Finding The Source of Medical Information

A Thesaurus-Index
to the
Reference Collection

Compiled by
BARBARA SMITH SHEARER
and **GENEVA L. BUSH**

Greenwood Press
Westport, Connecticut • London, England

Library of Congress Cataloging in Publication Data

Shearer, Barbara Smith.
  Finding the source of medical information.

  Includes index.
  1. Medicine—Bibliography. 2. Reference books—
Medicine—Bibliography. 3. Reference books—Medicine—
Indexes. I. Bush, Geneva L. II. Title. [DNLM:
1. Bibliography of Medicine. 2. Information Services.
3. Reference Books, Medical—bibliography.
ZWB 100 S539f]
Z6658.S4 1985 [R129]   016.61   84-22474
ISBN 0-313-24094-9 (lib. bdg.)

Library of Congress Catalog Card Number: 84-22474
ISBN: 0-313-24094-9

First published in 1985

Greenwood Press
A division of Congressional Information Service, Inc.
88 Post Road West, Westport, Connecticut 06881

Printed in the United States of America

10 9 8 7 6 5 4 3 2 1

To Ben, Tom, and Judy for listening

To Mom and Granny B. for understanding

CONTENTS

Preface ix

Acknowledgments xi

Introduction xiii

Citations 3

Alternate Title Index 35

Author Index 37

Thesaurus-Index 43

PREFACE

Though reference philosophies and methods differ broadly from
one library setting to another and from one librarian to another, the basic functions of a reference department remain the
same: to provide a well-balanced core reference collection; to
provide access to the core collection; and to provide trained
personnel for the retrieval of pertinent and accurate information.
        Efficient core collection development hinges on a clear
definition of the library's primary clientele and an understanding of the majority of the patrons' needs. Once this is
accomplished in a medical setting, one recognizes that the
highly specialized nature of the medical field requires a very
special kind of core collection. For instance, a great
percentage of medical reference is answered through the medical
journal literature and personal communication among health care
professionals. To gain access to the literature, and to sup-
plement state-of-the-art literature, once found, it is
necessary to turn to standard textbooks in each area of medical
specialization. This book is intended to aid in the delivery
of reference service by providing access to the books most
respected by the health care professionals themselves.
Traditional reference books such as directories, dictionaries,
and handbooks are still valid components of a medical reference
collection. In addition, reference materials designed for
different educational levels make medical literature more
accessible to nurses, technicians, students, laypersons, and
the beginning medical librarian, although none of the above may
be considered primary clientele.
        To date, no core list has been compiled that draws
together all levels and all types of medical reference and
textbook sources. Therefore, the first task in compiling this
book was to consult a variety of sources: comprehensive,
annotated bibliographies such as Chen's HEALTH SCIENCES
INFORMATION SOURCES, Lunin's HEALTH SCIENCES AND SERVICES,
Morton's USE OF MEDICAL LITERATURE (now entitled INFORMATION
SOURCES IN THE MEDICAL SCIENCES), and the Medical Library
Association's MEDICAL REFERENCE WORKS; handbooks for librarians

such as Darling's HANDBOOK OF MEDICAL LIBRARY PRACTICE and Roper and Boorkman's INTRODUCTION TO REFERENCE SOURCES IN THE HEALTH SCIENCES; specialized core collections appearing in journals such as the ANNALS OF INTERNAL MEDICINE's "Library for Internists, I-IV" and POSTGRADUATE MEDICINE's "Primary Care Physician's Book List"; and core lists of textbooks designed for specific types of libraries, such as the well-respected "Brandon lists" for small medical libraries and nursing collections. Altogether, over twenty lists were consulted and a core list developed with the assistance of, and recommendations from, medical librarians, physicians, pharmacists, and nurses. The final list is comprised primarily of medical books with a basic coverage in the areas of nursing and the allied health sciences, patient education, dentistry, and veterinary medicine.

As in FINDING THE SOURCE: A THESAURUS-INDEX TO THE REFERENCE COLLECTION (Benjamin F. Shearer and Barbara S. Shearer, Greenwood Press, 1981), the intent of this book is to provide a common-sense, natural language index to the contents of the core collection. The FINDING THE SOURCE idea was born out of frustration with using the artificial and confusing language of the Library of Congress Subject Headings as a means toward answering reference questions. Medical Subject Headings (MeSH), the counterpart designed by the National Library of Medicine, is indispensible for literature searching and subject cataloging within broad categories, but it is of little use with specific medical reference questions. By using the thesaurus terms (broader terms, narrower terms, and related terms), it is only a matter of one or two steps to pinpoint books containing the information sought. Call numbers may be penciled in to the left of the entry numbers in the first section of the book. This will allow the librarian to bypass the card catalog completely and go directly from FINDING THE SOURCE OF MEDICAL INFORMATION to the collection.

Finally, the trained medical librarian is not always available. It takes time and familiarity with medical literature and terminology to develop the skills required for the retrieval of accurate and pertinent information. Hopefully, this book will ease the strain of the transition to the medical field experienced by a beginning medical librarian, and will aid the more-seasoned reference librarian in gaining quick and efficient access to the reference collection.

ACKNOWLEDGMENTS

This project could never have been completed without the
combined efforts of many people.   The Medical Library
Association graciously allowed us to use Brandon and Hill's
"Selected List of Books and Journals for the Small Medical
Library" as part of a national survey of medical librarians.
The medical librarians themselves were most helpful in
completing the survey and in some cases took the time to
compile extensive lists of core reference books.
Recommendations of private physicians in Mobile and faculty
members at the University of South Alabama College of Medicine
were invaluable in making final decisions on specialty
textbooks for inclusion in our list.   Dr. Tim Martin, Clinical
Pharmacist at Mobile Infirmary, was most helpful in the areas
of pharmacology and toxicology.   The computer played a major
role in streamlining the indexing process.   We cannot
adequately express our gratitude for the generosity of Dr.
Charles Lowry for use of the computer and software, the
programming expertise of Andy Lightbourne, the ingenuity of
Sally Brennan, the helpfulness of Sonia Bishop, and the support
of our friends and colleagues at the University of South
Alabama.

INTRODUCTION

HOW TO USE THIS BOOK

FINDING THE SOURCE OF MEDICAL INFORMATION consists of two sections: bibliographic citations to 447 reference books and textbooks, and a thesaurus-index to the contents of the books cited. The citations are listed in alphabetical order by title with indexes for authors and alternate titles at the end of the citation section. Each bibliographic citation is given a distinct entry number further cited in the thesaurus-index. Section two combines the concept of thesaurus-building and detailed subject-indexing in a thesaurus-index. Every book cited in section one is indexed in multiple natural language terms or descriptors. The terms are matched with the entry numbers of the appropriate citations in section one. The following abbreviations are used throughout the thesaurus-index to describe the hierarchical relationships of descriptors: UF-Used For; BT-Broader Term; NT-Narrower Term; and RT-Related Term. The word "see" is employed to refer from a term not used for indexing to the preferred term used.

A strict thesaurus style was not possible due to the complexities of the subject matter and the combination of reference books and textbooks used for a core list. For example, "Skin" contains a "see" reference to "Dermatology," and though the relationship is not one usually found in a thesaurus, one is led to the appropriate term for discussions of all aspects of skin care, skin diseases, skin anatomy, etc. The manageable size of the core collection made it possible to construct the thesaurus with a very practical approach to the actual contents of the core collection as a whole.

In addition, the provision of multiple tiers used extensively throughout the thesaurus allowed for a conceptually thorough index to the core collection. A case by case determination was made regarding the most appropriate hierarchy of terms within each thesaurus entry. For effective use of the index, it is necessary to scan the entire thesaurus entry before going on to another thesaurus access point. Using cross

references and other index terms found beneath thesaurus
entries as additional entry points and scanning nearby
thesaurus entries as one would do in any other index will
further enhance its effectiveness. Not all index terms under
thesaurus entries are themselves thesaurus entries since this
would have made the index much too cumbersome. However, an
effort was made to include as many access points as possible
while maintaining control over the vocabulary.

There are two approaches to the contents of the core
collection: by subject, and by type of information. It is
best to go to the most specific term first and proceed with the
suggestions mentioned above for obtaining additional thesaurus
access points. Sometimes, and especially for the beginning
medical librarian, groundwork is necessary. Fortunately, this
is very simple to do. A good, basic medical dictionary such as
Miller and Keane's ENCYCLOPEDIA AND DICTIONARY OF MEDICINE,
NURSING, AND ALLIED HEALTH will help in defining and
classifying a reference question. Once this is accomplished,
there are several special categories in the thesaurus that
provide a sizable number of the total subject entries. An
example is the term "Diseases." Specific names of diseases are
not listed as thesaurus entries with the exception of the
narrower terms mentioned under the entry "Diseases." Instead,
"Diseases" indicates the books that cover specific diseases and
the term will be found elsewhere in the thesaurus-index under
the body system most affected or by the medical specialty most
often called upon to treat the disease. If the subject
approach does not succeed initially, a quick look at the
"Diseases" entry will provide the user with possible terms for
direct subject access. Other thesaurus entries with similar
applications are "Pediatrics," "Treatment," "Drugs,"
"Directories," "Nursing Practice," and "Patient Education."
The latter two terms have been used as designations for nursing
and consumer oriented books in the core collection. They can
be used by public libraries as well as medical libraries for
consumer collection development purposes and as entry points
for the unsophisticated user. "Drugs (Treatment Modality)" is
used for specialty textbooks that include major sections
discussing drug therapy for specific diseases or types of
diseases.

The scope of this book is the United States. However, a
few directories include Canada, the United Kingdom, Europe, or
are international in scope. This is often indicated in the
title of the book. In addition, there are separate entries,
"Canada" and "United Kingdom," established for books
specifically covering those geographic areas.

The following sample search explains how to use the
thesaurus-index effectively.

"WHAT ARE THE SIGNS AND SYMPTOMS OF FOOD POISONING?"

Step 1. Choose the most particular word or words of this question.

The two major elements of this question are "food
poisoning" and "signs and symptoms." The most specific
approach is "food poisoning."

FOOD POISONING

> BT Poisoning
> Complications 259
> Control 259
> Diagnosis 168, 193, 259
> Epidemiology 259
> Etiology 259
> History 259
> Immunology 259
> Nursing practice 144
> Occurrence 259
> Pathology 259
> Prevention 193, 259
> Prognosis 193
> Signs and symptoms 168,
> 193, 259
> Transmission 259
> Treatment 168, 193, 259

Note that three sources provide signs and symptoms of food poisoning.

Step 2. Find entry numbers 168, 193, and 259 in section one.

168. Gastroenterology, edited by Henry L. Bockus, et al. 3rd ed. Philadelphia: Saunders, 1974-1976. (4v.)

193. Handbook of poisoning: prevention, diagnosis & treatment, by Robert H. Dreisbach. 11th ed. Los Altos, CA: Lange, 1983.

259. Maxcy-Rosenau public health and preventive medicine, edited by John M. Last. 11th ed. New York: Appleton-Century-Crofts, 1980.

At this point, it might be to the user's advantage to go ahead and check the broader term "Poisoning." The three sources listed above would have probably answered the question. However, if the patient involved is a child, the section from the thesaurus entry "Poisoning" may have been of interest.

POISONING

> NT Food poisoning
> RT Bites and stings
> RT Emergency care
> .
> .
> .
> Pediatrics
>   Etiology 195
>   Signs and symptoms 192,
>   195, 304
>   Treatment 108, 109,
>   192, 195, 304

Note that three additional books were located on poisoning (probably with sections on food poisoning) specifically in pediatrics.

192.   Handbook of pediatrics, by Henry K. Silver, et al. 14th ed. Los Altos, CA: Lange, 1983.

195.   Harriet Lane handbook: a manual for pediatric house officers, edited by Jeffrey A. Biller and Andrew M. Yeager. 9th ed. Chicago: Year Book, 1981.

304.   Nelson textbook of pediatrics, by Richard E. Behrman and Victor C. Vaughan, III. 12th ed. Philadelphia: Saunders, 1983.

The term "Signs and symptoms" is also a thesaurus entry and the same information could have been located by going there first. However, the multiple tiers make it more difficult to use than the direct subject approach.

"Food poisoning" is a very straightforward topic for a reference question and there was no need to conceptualize before using the thesaurus. However, there are many cases where it is necessary to classify a disease or disorder before proceeding. For instance, if one wants signs and symptoms of an ulcer, it is essential to know that an ulcer affects the gastrointestinal system. "Gastrointestinal system" is a thesaurus entry while "ulcer" is not.

Clearly, not all aspects of any one given source are indexed in this book. However, the ability to conceptualize topics is learned over a period of time. As one gains experience in using traditional reference sources and in viewing textbooks as valuable reference sources, the index will change roles. At first, it is hoped that this book will serve as an introduction to the core medical reference books. Eventually, the experienced reference librarian will want to use it as a ready reference handbook to the core collection.

Nurses, nursing students, technicians, and laypersons who often want to gain access to the medical literature for further study will be able to start at a more basic level and proceed to the specialty textbooks. Physicians who are quite familiar with the names of their favorite textbooks may need help with other specialty texts. Finally, medical students have a need for rapid familiarity with all specialty textbooks. FINDING THE SOURCE OF MEDICAL INFORMATION will provide them with a list and the means to become quickly oriented to core medical literature.

Finding
the Source
of Medical
Information

CITATIONS

1. AAMC curriculum directory. Washington, DC: Association of American Medical Colleges, 1973--. (annual)

2. AAMC directory of American medical education.
   Washington, DC: Association of American Medical
   Colleges, 1969--. (annual)

3. Abbreviations in medicine, by Edwin B. Steen. 4th ed.
   New York: Macmillan, 1978.

4. Abdominal operations, by Rodney Maingot. 7th ed. New
   York: Appleton-Century-Crofts, 1980. (2v.)

5. Accepted dental therapeutics. Chicago: American Dental
   Association, 1934--. (biennial)

6. Accreditation manual for hospitals. Chicago: Joint
   Commission on Accreditation of Hospitals, 1969--.
   (annual)

7. Ackerman and del Regato's cancer: diagnosis, treatment,
   and prognosis, by Juan A. del Regato and Harlan J.
   Spjut. 5th ed. St. Louis: Mosby, 1977.

8. Ackerman's surgical pathology, by Juan Rosai. 6th ed.
   St. Louis: Mosby, 1981. (2v.)

9. Acronyms, initialisms, and abbreviations dictionary,
   edited by Ellen T. Crowley. 8th ed. Detroit: Gale,
   1983--. (3v.)

10. Admission requirements of U.S. and Canadian dental
    schools. Washington, DC: American Association of
    Dental Schools, 1965--. (annual)

11. Alexander's care of the patient in surgery, by Barbara J.
     Gruendemann and Margaret Huth Meeker. 7th ed. St.
     Louis: Mosby, 1983.

12. Allergy: principles and practice, edited by Elliott
     Middleton, Jr., et al. 2nd ed. St. Louis: Mosby,
     1983. (2v.)

13. Allied health education directory. Chicago: American
     Medical Association, 1978--. (annual)

14. AMA directory of officials and staff. Chicago: American
     Medical Association, 1979--.

15. AMA drug evaluations, by the American Medical Associa-
     tion. 5th ed. Philadelphia: Saunders, 1983.

16. American College of Surgeons: 1983 yearbook. Chicago:
     The College, 1983.

17. American dental directory. Chicago: American Dental
     Association, 1947--. (annual)

18. American drug index, by Norman F. Billups and Shirley M.
     Billups. 28th ed. Philadelphia: Lippincott, 1984.

19. American druggist blue book. New York: Hearst, 1928--.
     (annual)

20. American hospital formulary service drug information.
     Bethesda, MD: American Society of Hospital Pharma-
     cists, 1984--. (annual with quarterly supplements)

21. American Medical Association family medical guide, by
     Jeffrey R. M. Kunz. New York: Random, 1982.

22. American medical directory. Chicago: American Medical
     Association, 1906--.

23. American men and women of science. Physical & biological
     sciences. 15th ed. New York: Bowker, 1982.

24. Anatomy for surgeons, by W. Henry Hollinshead. 2nd ed.
     Philadelphia: Harper & Row, 1968-1971. (3v.) (3rd ed.,
     1982--.)

25. Anatomy of the human body, edited by Charles Mayo Goss;
     with new drawings by Don M. Alvarado. 29th ed.
     Philadelphia: Lea & Febiger, 1973.

26. Andrews' diseases of the skin: clinical dermatology, by
     Anthony N. Domonkos, et al. 7th ed. Philadelphia:
     Saunders, 1982.

27. Anesthesia, edited by Ronald D. Miller. New York:
     Churchill Livingstone, 1981. (2v.)

28. Anesthesia and uncommon diseases: pathophysiologic and
    clinical correlations, by Jordan Katz, et al. 2nd ed.
    Philadelphia: Saunders, 1981.

29. Anesthesia for infants and children, by Robert M. Smith.
    4th ed. St. Louis: Mosby, 1980.

30. Applied therapeutics: the clinical use of drugs, edited
    by Brian S. Katcher, et al. 3rd ed. San Francisco:
    Applied Therapeutics, 1983.

31. Arthritis and allied conditions: a textbook of
    rheumatology, edited by Daniel J. McCarty. 9th ed.
    Philadelphia: Lea & Febiger, 1979.

32. Atlas of head and neck surgery, by John M. Lore. 2nd ed.
    Philadelphia: Saunders, 1973. (2v.)

33. Atlas of human histology, by Mariano S. H. di Fiore. 5th
    ed. Philadelphia: Lea & Febiger, 1981.

34. Author's guide to journals in nursing & related fields,
    edited by Steven D. Warner and Kathryn D. Schweer. New
    York: Haworth, 1982.

35. Bailey and Scott's diagnostic microbiology, by Sydney M.
    Finegold and William J. Martin. 6th ed. St. Louis:
    Mosby, 1982.

36. Barron's guide to medical & dental schools, by Saul
    Wischnitzer. Woodbury, NY: Barron's Educational
    Series, 1982.

37. Basic and clinical immunology, edited by Daniel P. Stites,
    et al. Los Altos, CA: Lange, 1976--. (biennial)

38. Bedside diagnostic examination, by Elmer L. DeGowin and
    Richard L. DeGowin. 4th ed. New York: Macmillan,
    1981.

39. Bergey's manual of determinative bacteriology, edited by
    R. E. Buchanan and N. E. Gibbons. 8th ed. Baltimore:
    Williams & Wilkins, 1974. (9th ed., 1984--.)

40. Best and Taylor's physiological basis of medical
    practice, edited by John B. West. 11th ed. Baltimore:
    Williams & Wilkins, 1984.

41. Bibliography of bioethics. Detroit: Gale, 1975--.

42. Bibliography of the history of medicine. Bethesda, MD:
    National Library of Medicine, 1965--. (annual)

43. Biochemistry: the molecular basis of cell structure and
    function, by Albert L. Lehninger. 3rd ed. New York:
    Worth, 1983.

44. Biographical directory: fellows and members of the
     American Psychiatric Association as of January 1983.
     Washington, DC: American Psychiatric Association,
     1983.

45. Biographical directory of the American College of
     Physicians, 1979. New York: Jaques Cattell Press,
     Bowker, 1979.

46. Biographical directory of the American Public Health
     Association. New York: Jaques Cattell Press, Bowker,
     1979.

47. A Biographical history of medicine: excerpts and essays
     on the men and their work, by John H. Talbott. New
     York: Grune & Stratton, 1970.

48. Biology data book, edited by Philip L. Altman and Dorothy
     S. Dittmer. 2nd ed. Bethesda, MD: Federation of
     American Societies for Experimental Biology, 1972-1974.
     (3v.)

49. Birth defects compendium, edited by Daniel Bergsma. 2nd
     ed. New York: published for the National Foundation-
     March of Dimes by A. R. Liss, 1979.

50. Black's medical dictionary, by William A. R. Thomson.
     33rd ed. Totowa, NJ: Barnes & Noble, 1981.

51. Black's veterinary dictionary, edited by Geoffrey P.
     West. 14th rev. ed. Totowa, NJ: Barnes & Noble,
     1982.

52. Blakiston's Gould medical dictionary, edited by Alfonso
     R. Gennaro, et al. 4th ed. New York: McGraw-Hill,
     1979.

53. Books in print. New York: Bowker, 1948--. (annual)

54. Bowes and Church's food values of portions commonly used,
     revised by Jean A. T. Pennington and Helen Nichols
     Church. 13th ed. Philadelphia: Lippincott, 1980.

55. British pharmacopoeia. London: Pharmaceutical Press,
     1864--.

56. Campbell's operative orthopedics, edited by Allen S.
     Edmonson and A. H. Crenshaw. 6th ed. St. Louis:
     Mosby, 1980. (2v.)

57. Campbell's urology, edited by J. Hartwell Harrison, et
     al. 4th ed. Philadelphia: Saunders, 1978-1979. (3v.)

58. Canadian hospital directory. Toronto: Canadian Hospital
     Association, 1953--.

59. Cancer facts and figures. New York: American Cancer
       Society, 1983.

60. Cancer medicine, edited by James F. Holland and Emil
       Frei, III. 2nd ed. Philadelphia: Lea & Febiger,
       1982.

61. Cancer: principles and practice of oncology, edited by
       Vincent T. DeVita, et al. Philadelphia: Lippincott,
       1982.

62. Cardiac nursing, by Sandra L. Underhill, et al. Phila-
       delphia: Lippincott, 1982.

63. Carini and Owens' neurological and neurosurgical nursing,
       by Barbara Lang Conway-Rutkowski. 8th ed. St. Louis:
       Mosby, 1982.

64. Catalog of teratogenic agents, by Thomas H. Shepard. 4th
       ed. Baltimore: Johns Hopkins University Press, 1983.

65. Catalogue of strains I. Rockville, MD: American Type
       Culture Collection, 1976--. (biennial)

66. Catalogue of strains II. Rockville, MD: American Type
       Culture Collection, 1975--. (biennial)

67. Cecil textbook of medicine, edited by James B. Wyngaarden
       and Lloyd H. Smith, Jr. 16th ed. Philadelphia:
       Saunders, 1982.

68. Chem sources--U.S.A. Ormond Beach, FL: Directories
       Publishing, 1973--. (annual)

69. Chromosomal variation in man: a catalog of chromosomal
       variants and anomalies, by Digamber S. Borgaonkar. 4th
       ed. New York: A. R. Liss, 1984.

70. Ciba collection of medical illustrations, prepared by
       Frank H. Netter. West Caldwell, NJ: Ciba
       Pharmaceutical Co., 1983--.

71. Classic descriptions of disease: with biographical
       sketches of the authors, by Ralph H. Major. 3rd ed.
       Springfield, IL: Thomas, 1945.

72. Clinical aspects of aging: a comprehensive text prepared
       under the direction of the American Geriatrics Society,
       edited by William Reichel. 2nd ed. Baltimore:
       Williams & Wilkins, 1983.

73. Clinical aspects of immunology, edited by P. J. Lachmann
       and D. K. Peters. 4th ed. St. Louis: Mosby, 1982.
       (2v.)

74. Clinical disorders of fluid and electrolyte metabolism,
     edited by Morton H. Maxwell and Charles R. Kleeman.
     3rd ed. New York: McGraw-Hill, 1980.

75. Clinical gastroenterology, by Howard M. Spiro. 3rd ed.
     New York: Macmillan, 1983.

76. Clinical gynecologic endocrinology and infertility, by
     Leon Speroff, et al. 3rd ed. Baltimore: Williams &
     Wilkins, 1983.

77. Clinical hematology, by Maxwell M. Wintrobe, et al. 8th
     ed. Philadelphia: Lea & Febiger, 1981.

78. Clinical hypertension, by Norman M. Kaplan. 3rd ed.
     Baltimore: Williams & Wilkins, 1982.

79. Clinical interpretation and practice of cancer chemo-
     therapy, edited by Ezra M. Greenspan. New York:
     Raven, 1982.

80. Clinical interpretation of laboratory tests, by Frances
     K. Widmann. 9th ed. Philadelphia: Davis, 1983.

81. Clinical medicine, edited by John A. Spittell, et al.
     Rev. ed. Philadelphia: Harper & Row, 1983--. (loose-
     leaf) (12v.)

82. Clinical neurology, edited by A. B. Baker and L. H.
     Baker. Rev. ed. Philadelphia: Harper & Row, 1983--.
     (loose-leaf) (4v.)

83. Clinical parasitology, by Paul Chester Beaver, et al.
     9th ed. Philadelphia: Lea & Febiger, 1984.

84. Clinical rheumatology: a problem-oriented approach to
     diagnosis and management, by Roland W. Moskowitz. 2nd
     ed. Philadelphia: Lea & Febiger, 1982.

85. Clinical toxicology of commercial products, by Robert E.
     Gosselin, et al. 4th ed. Baltimore: Williams &
     Wilkins, 1976.

86. Community cancer programs in the United States: the
     delegates roster of the Association of Community Cancer
     Centers. Washington, DC: The Association, 1980--.
     (annual)

87. Compilation of experimental cancer therapy protocol
     summaries. 7th ed. Rockville, MD: National
     Institutes of Health, 1983.

88. Comprehensive pediatric nursing, edited by Gladys M.
     Scipien, et al. 2nd ed. New York: McGraw-Hill,
     1979.

89. Comprehensive textbook of psychiatry III, edited by
     Harold I. Kaplan, et al. 3rd ed. Baltimore:
     Williams & Wilkins, 1980. (3v.)

90. Consumer health information source book, by Alan M. Rees
     and Blanche A. Young. New York: Bowker, 1981.

91. Control of communicable diseases in man: an official
     report of the American Public Health Association,
     edited by Abram S. Benenson. 13th ed. Washington,
     DC: The Association, 1981.

92. Correlative neuroanatomy & functional neurology, by
     Joseph G. Chusid. Los Altos, CA: Lange, 1952--.
     (triennial)

93. CRC composite index for CRC handbooks. 2nd ed. Cleve-
     land: CRC Press, 1977.

94. CRC handbook of biochemistry and molecular biology,
     edited by Gerald D. Fasman. 3rd ed. Cleveland: CRC
     Press, 1975-1977. (Section A: Proteins; Section B:
     Nucleic acids; Section C: Lipids, carbohydrates,
     steroids; Section D: Physical and chemical data)

95. CRC handbook of chemistry and physics. Boca Raton, FL:
     CRC Press, 1914--. (annual)

96. CRC handbook of engineering in medicine and biology,
     edited by David G. Fleming and Barry N. Feinberg.
     Cleveland: CRC Press, 1976-1978.

97. CRC handbook of laboratory animal science, by Edward C.
     Melby and Norman H. Altman. Cleveland: CRC Press,
     1974-1976. (3v.)

98. CRC handbook of microbiology, edited by Allen I. Laskin
     and Hubert A. Lechevalier. 2nd ed. Cleveland; Boca
     Raton, FL: CRC Press, 1977-1982. (v. 1: Bacteria; v.
     2: Fungi, algae, protozoa, and viruses; v. 3:
     Microbial composition: amino acids, proteins, and
     nucleic acids; v. 4: Microbial composition: carbo-
     hydrates, lipids, and minerals)

99. CRC handbook series in clinical laboratory science,
     edited by David Seligson. Cleveland; Boca Raton, FL:
     CRC Press, 1977-1982. (Section A: Nuclear medicine;
     Section B: Toxicology; Section C: Pathology; Section
     D: Blood banking; Section E: Clinical microbiology;
     Section F: Immunology; Section G: Clinical chemis-
     try; Section H: Virology & rickettsiology; Section I:
     Hematology)

100. Critical care nursing, edited by Carolyn M. Hudak, et
     al. 3rd ed. Philadelphia: Lippincott, 1982.

101.   Current clinical dental terminology, edited by Carl O.
        Boucher. 3rd ed. St. Louis: Mosby, 1982.

102.   Current contents: clinical practice. Philadelphia:
        Institute for Scientific Information, 1973--. (weekly)

103.   Current contents: life sciences. Philadelphia:
        Institute for Scientific Information, 1967--. (weekly)

104.   Current diagnosis 6, edited by Howard F. Conn and Rex B.
        Conn, Jr. Philadelphia: Saunders, 1980.

105.   Current medical diagnosis & treatment, edited by Marcus
        A. Krupp and Milton J. Chatton. Los Altos, CA:
        Lange, 1974--. (annual)

106.   Current obstetric & gynecologic diagosis & treatment,
        edited by Ralph C. Benson. Los Altos, CA: Lange,
        1976--. (biennial)

107.   Current operative urology, edited by E. Douglas
        Whitehead and Elliot Leiter. 2nd ed. Philadelphia:
        Lippincott, 1984.

108.   Current pediatric diagnosis & treatment, edited by C.
        Henry Kempe, et al. Los Altos, CA: Lange, 1970--.
        (biennial)

109.   Current pediatric therapy, edited by Sydney S. Gellis
        and Benjamin M. Kagan. Philadelphia: Saunders,
        1964--. (biennial)

110.   Current surgical diagnosis & treatment, edited by
        Lawrence W. Way. Los Altos, CA: Lange, 1973--.
        (biennial)

111.   Current therapy, edited by Robert E. Rakel. Philadel-
        phia: Saunders, 1949--. (annual)

112.   Current urologic therapy, edited by Joseph J. Kaufman.
        Philadelphia: Saunders, 1980.

113.   Current veterinary therapy, edited by R. W. Kirk.
        Philadelphia: Saunders, 1965--.

114.   Dangerous properties of industrial materials, by N.
        Irving Sax. 5th ed. New York: Van Nostrand, 1979.

115.   De Palma's the management of fractures and dislocations:
        an atlas, edited by John F. Connolly. 3rd ed.
        Philadelphia: Saunders, 1981. (2v.)

116.   Dermatology in general medicine: textbook and atlas,
        edited by Thomas B. Fitzpatrick, et al. 2nd ed. New
        York: McGraw-Hill, 1979. (1983 Update)

117. Diagnosis of diseases of the chest, by Robert G. Fraser
     and J. A. Peter Pare. 2nd ed. Philadelphia:
     Saunders, 1977-1979. (4v.)

118. Diagnostic and statistical manual of mental disorders.
     3rd ed. Washington, DC: American Psychiatric
     Association, 1980.

119. Dictionary of abbreviations in medicine and the health
     sciences, by Harold K. Hughes. Lexington, MA:
     Lexington Books, 1977.

120. Dictionary of health services management, edited by
     Thomas Timmreck. Owings Mills, MD: National Health
     Publishing, 1982.

121. Dictionary of medical syndromes, by Sergio I. Magalini
     and Euclide Scrascia. 2nd ed. Philadelphia:
     Lippincott, 1981.

122. Differential diagnosis: the interpretation of clinical
     evidence, by A. McGehee Harvey, et al. 3rd ed.
     Philadelphia: Saunders, 1979.

123. Directory American College of Hospital Administrators:
     a biographical dictionary of the membership. Chicago:
     The College, 1981.

124. Directory of directories, edited by J. M. Ethridge and
     C. A. Marlow. Detroit: Information Enterprises;
     distributed by Gale, 1980--. (biennial with
     supplements)

125. Directory of health science libraries in the United
     States, 1979, edited by Alan M. Rees and Susan
     Crawford, with the assistance of Margaret Henning.
     Cleveland: Cleveland Health Sciences Library of Case
     Western Reserve University; Chicago: distributed by
     Medical Library Association, 1980.

126. Directory of medical specialists. Chicago: published
     for the American Board of Medical Specialties by
     Marquis Who's Who, 1975--. (biennial)

127. Directory of published proceedings: series SEMT--
     science/engineering/medicine/technology. Harrison,
     NY: InterDok, 1965--. (monthly with annual
     cumulation)

128. Directory of residency training programs accredited by
     the Accreditation Council for Graduate Medical
     Education. Chicago: American Medical Association,
     1979--. (annual)

129. Directory of special libraries and information centers,
      edited by Brigitte T. Darnay and Sharon L. Stanton.
      8th ed. Detroit: Gale, 1983. (supplemented by New
      special libraries)

130. Directory of women physicians in the U.S. 2nd ed.
      Chicago: American Medical Association, 1979.

131. Diseases of exotic animals: medical and surgical manage-
      ment, by Joel D. Wallach and William J. Boever.
      Philadelphia: Saunders, 1983.

132. Diseases of the liver, edited by Leon Schiff and Eugene
      R. Schiff. 5th ed. Philadelphia: Lippincott, 1982.

133. Diseases of the liver and biliary system, by Sheila
      Sherlock. 6th ed. St. Louis: Mosby, 1981.

134. Dorland's illustrated medical dictionary. 26th ed.
      Philadelphia: Saunders, 1981.

135. Drug interactions: clinical significance of drug-drug
      interactions and drug effects on clinical laboratory
      results, by Philip D. Hansten. 4th ed. Philadelphia:
      Lea & Febiger, 1979.

136. Drug topics red book: annual pharmacists' reference.
      Oradell, NJ: Medical Economics, 1857--. (annual)

137. Drugs and nursing implications, by Laura E. Govoni and
      Janice E. Hayes. 4th ed. Norwalk, CT: Appleton-
      Century-Crofts, 1982.

138. Drugs in current use and new drugs, edited by Walter
      Modell. New York: Springer, 1955--. (annual)

139. Drugs of choice, edited by Walter Modell. St. Louis:
      Mosby, 1959--. (biennial)

140. Echocardiography, by Harvey Feigenbaum. 3rd ed.
      Philadelphia: Lea & Febiger, 1981.

141. Elsevier's medical dictionary in five languages:
      English/American, French, Italian, Spanish and German,
      by A. Sliosberg. 2nd rev. ed. Amsterdam, New York:
      Elsevier Scientific Publishing, 1975.

142. Emergency medicine: a comprehensive review, edited by
      Thomas Clarke Kravis and Carmen Germaine Warner.
      Rockville, MD: Aspen, 1983.

143. Emergency medicine: concepts and clinical practice, by
      Peter Rosen, et al. St. Louis: Mosby, 1983. (2v.)

144. Emergency nursing: principles and practice, by Susan A.
      Budassi and Janet M. Barber. St. Louis: Mosby, 1981.

145. Encyclopedia and dictionary of medicine, nursing, and
      allied health, by Benjamin F. Miller and Claire Brack-
      man Keane. 3rd ed. Philadelphia: Saunders, 1983.

146. Encyclopedia of animal care, edited by Geoffrey P. West.
      12th ed. Baltimore: Williams & Wilkins, 1977.

147. Encyclopedia of associations. Detroit: Gale, 1961--.
      (annual)

148. Encyclopedia of bioethics, edited by Warren T. Reich.
      New York: Free Press, 1978. (4v.)

149. Encyclopedia of common natural ingredients used in food,
      drugs, and cosmetics, by Albert Y. Leung. New York:
      Wiley, 1980.

150. Encyclopedia of information systems and services, edited
      by John Schmittroth, Jr., et al. 5th ed. Detroit:
      Gale, 1983. (supplemented by New information systems
      and services)

151. Encyclopedia of medical organizations and agencies,
      edited by Anthony T. Kruzas. Detroit: Gale, 1983--.
      (annual)

152. Encyclopedia of medical sources, by Emerson Crosby
      Kelly. Baltimore: Williams & Wilkins, 1948.

153. Endocrinology, edited by Leslie J. DeGroot, et al. New
      York: Grune & Stratton, 1979. (3v.)

154. Enzyme nomenclature, 1978: recommendations of the
      Nomenclature Committee of the International Union of
      Biochemistry on the Nomenclature and Classification of
      Enzymes. New York: published for the Union by
      Academic Press, 1979.

155. European pharmacopoeia, published under the direction of
      the Council of Europe (partial agreement) in
      accordance with the Convention on the Elaboration of a
      European Pharmacopoeia. 2nd ed. Sainte-Ruffine,
      France: Maisonneuve, 1980.

156. Evaluations of drug interactions. 2nd ed. Washington,
      DC: American Pharmaceutical Association, 1976.

157. Facts about nursing. Kansas City, MO: American Nurses'
      Association, 1935--. (annual)

158. Facts and comparisons. St. Louis: Facts and Compari-
      sons, 1979--. (loose-leaf) (2v.)

159.   Facts at your fingertips: a guide to sources of statis-
        tical information on major health topics. Hyatts-
        ville: National Center for Health Statistics, 1978--.

160.   Falconer's the drug, the nurse, the patient, including
        Current drug handbook, 1982-84, by Eleanor Sheridan,
        et al. 7th ed. Philadelphia: Saunders, 1982.

161.   Familiar medical quotations, edited by Maurice B.
        Strauss. Boston: Little, Brown, 1968.

162.   Finding the source: a thesaurus-index to the reference
        collection, by Benjamin F. Shearer and Barbara Smith
        Shearer. Westport, CT: Greenwood, 1981.

163.   Foundation directory, edited by Loren Renz, et al.   9th
        ed. New York: Foundation Center; distributed by
        Columbia University Press, 1983.

164.   Foundation grants index. New York: Foundation Center;
        distributed by Columbia University Press, 1971--.
        (bimonthly with annual cumulation)

165.   Fractures, edited by Charles A. Rockwood, Jr., et al.
        Philadelphia: Lippincott, 1984. (3v.: Fractures in
        adults and Fractures in children)

166.   French's index of differential diagnosis, edited by F.
        Dudley Hart. 11th ed. Chicago: John Wright;
        distributed by Year Book, 1979.

167.   Fundamentals of nursing practice, by Barbara W. Narrow
        and Kay Brown Buschle. New York: Wiley, 1982.

168.   Gastroenterology, edited by Henry L. Bockus, et al.   3rd
        ed. Philadelphia: Saunders, 1974-1976. (4v.)

169.   Gastrointestinal disease: pathophysiology, diagnosis,
        management, edited by Marvin H. Sleisenger and John S.
        Fordtran. 3rd ed. Philadelphia: Saunders, 1983.

170.   Geigy scientific tables, edited by C. Lentner. 8th rev.
        and enl. ed. West Caldwell, NJ: Ciba-Geigy, 1981--.

171.   General ophthalmology, by Daniel Vaughan, et al. Los
        Altos, CA: Lange, 1958--. (triennial)

172.   General urology, by Donald R. Smith. Los Altos, CA:
        Lange, 1957--. (triennial)

173.   Gibbon's surgery of the chest, edited by David C.
        Sabiston, Jr. and Frank C. Spencer. 4th ed. Phila-
        delphia: Saunders, 1983. (2v.)

174.   Golden's diagnostic radiology, series edited by Laurence
        L. Robbins. Baltimore: Williams & Wilkins, 1980--.

175. Goodman and Gilman's the pharmacological basis of thera-
      peutics, edited by Alfred Goodman Gilman, et. al. 6th
      ed. New York: Macmillan, 1980.

176. Gourman report: a rating of graduate and professional
      programs in American and international universities,
      by Jack Gourman. 2nd rev. ed. Los Angeles: National
      Education Standards, 1983.

177. Gourman report: a rating of undergraduate programs in
      American and international universities, by Jack
      Gourman. 4th rev. ed. Los Angeles: National Educa-
      tion Standards, 1983.

178. Graduate medical education announcements, by William E.
      Briggs, et al. Columbus, OH: Major Hospital Atlas,
      1974--. (annual)

179. Gradwohl's clinical laboratory methods and diagnosis: a
      textbook on laboratory procedures and their interpre-
      tation, edited by Alex C. Sonnenwirth and Leonard
      Jarett. 8th ed. St. Louis: Mosby, 1980. (2v.)

180. Grant's atlas of anatomy, by James E. Anderson. 8th ed.
      Baltimore: Williams & Wilkins, 1983.

181. A Guide to physical examination, by Barbara Bates. 3rd
      ed. Philadelphia: Lippincott, 1983.

182. Guide to reference books, by Eugene P. Sheehy, with the
      assistance of Rita G. Keckeissen and Eileen McIlvaine.
      9th ed. Chicago: American Library Association, 1976.
      (2 supplements)

183. Guide to scientific instruments. Washington, DC:
      American Association for the Advancement of Science,
      1963--. (annual)

184. Guide to the health care field. Chicago: American
      Hospital Association, 1972--. (annual)

185. Gynecologic and obstetric urology, by Herbert J.
      Buchsbaum and Joseph D. Schmidt. 2nd ed. Philadel-
      phia: Saunders, 1982.

186. Gynecology of childhood and adolescence, by John W.
      Huffman, et al. 2nd ed. Philadelphia: Saunders,
      1981.

187. Handbook of clinical dietetics, by the American Dietetic
      Association. New Haven: Yale University Press, 1981.

188. Handbook of clinical drug data, edited by James E.
      Knoben, et al. 5th ed. Hamilton, IL: Drug Intelli-
      gence Publications, 1983.

189. Handbook of drug therapy in psychiatry, by Jerrold G.
      Bernstein. Boston: John Wright, 1983.

190. Handbook of nonprescription drugs. 7th ed. Washington,
      DC: American Pharmaceutical Association, 1982.

191. Handbook of obstetrics & gynecology, edited by Ralph C.
      Benson. Los Altos, CA: Lange, 1964--. (triennial)

192. Handbook of pediatrics, by Henry K. Silver, et al. 14th
      ed. Los Altos, CA: Lange, 1983.

193. Handbook of poisoning: prevention, diagnosis &
      treatment, by Robert H. Dreisbach. 11th ed. Los
      Altos, CA: Lange, 1983.

194. Handbook on injectable drugs, by Lawrence A. Trissel.
      3rd ed. Washington, DC: American Society of Hospital
      Pharmacists, 1983.

195. Harriet Lane handbook: a manual for pediatric house
      officers, edited by Jeffrey A. Biller and Andrew M.
      Yeager. 9th ed. Chicago: Year Book, 1981.

196. Harrison's principles of internal medicine, edited by
      Robert G. Petersdorf, et al. 10th ed. New York:
      McGraw-Hill, 1983.

197. Health care supervisor's handbook, by Norman Metzger.
      2nd ed. Rockville, MD: Aspen, 1982.

198. Health organizations of the United States, Canada and
      the world, by Paul Wasserman and Marek Kaszubski. 5th
      ed. Detroit: Gale, 1981.

199. Health resources statistics. Hyattsville, MD: National
      Center for Health Statistics, 1965--.

200. Health science books 1876-1982. New York: Bowker,
      1982. (4v.)

201. Health sciences information sources, by Ching-chih Chen.
      Cambridge, MA: Massachusetts Institute of Technology,
      1981.

202. Health sciences serials. Bethesda, MD: National
      Library of Medicine, 1979--. (microfiche) (quarterly)

203. Health services directory, edited by Anthony T. Kruzas,
      et al. Detroit: Gale, 1981.

204. Health: United States. Washington, DC: National
      Center for Health Statistics, 1975--. (annual)

205. Heart, arteries and veins, edited by J. Willis Hurst, et
      al. 5th ed. New York: McGraw-Hill, 1982. (2v.)

206. Heart disease: a textbook of cardiovascular medicine,
      edited by Eugene Braunwald. 2nd ed. Philadelphia:
      Saunders, 1984.

207. Hematology, edited by William J. Williams, et al. 3rd
      ed. New York: McGraw-Hill, 1983.

208. Hematology of infancy and childhood, edited by David G.
      Nathan and Frank A. Oski. 2nd ed. Phialdelphia:
      Saunders, 1981.

209. Henderson's dictionary of biological terms, by Sandra
      Holmes. 9th ed. New York: Van Nostrand, 1979.

210. Hospital dental practice, edited by James R. Hooley and
      Lowell G. Daun. St. Louis: Mosby, 1980.

211. Hospital literature index. Chicago: American Hospital
      Association, 1945--. (quarterly with annual
      cumulation)

212. Hospital statistics. Chicago: American Hospital
      Association, 1972--. (annual)

213. How to write and publish papers in the medical sciences,
      by Edward J. Huth. Philadelphia: Institute for
      Scientific Information, 1982.

214. Human sexuality in health and illness, by Nancy Fugate
      Woods. 3rd ed. St. Louis: Mosby, 1984.

215. Hunter's tropical medicine, edited by J. Thomas Strick-
      land. 6th ed. Philadelphia: Saunders, 1984.

216. Illustrated dictionary of dentistry, by Stanley
      Jablonski. Philadelphia: Saunders, 1982.

217. Illustrated dictionary of eponymic syndromes, by Stanley
      Jablonski. Philadelphia: Saunders, 1969.

218. Index medicus. Bethesda, MD: National Library of
      Medicine, 1960--. (monthly with annual cumulation)

219. Index of NLM serial titles. Bethesda, MD: National
      Library of Medicine, 1972--. (annual) (2v.)

220. Index of signs and symptoms of industrial diseases, by
      Betsy A. Fay and Charles E. Billings. Rockville, MD:
      National Institute for Occupational Safety and Health,
      1981. (index to Occupational diseases)

221. Index to scientific & technical proceedings. Phila-
      delphia: Institute for Scientific Information,
      1978--. (monthly with annual cumulation)

18   222. Index to scientific reviews

222.   Index to scientific reviews. Philadelphia: Institute
        for Scientific Information, 1978--. (semiannual) (2v.)

223.   Infectious diseases: a modern treatise of infectious
        processes, edited by Paul D. Hoeprich. 3rd ed.
        Philadelphia: Harper & Row, 1983.

224.   Infectious diseases of children, by Saul Krugman and
        Samuel L. Katz. 7th ed. St. Louis: Mosby, 1981.

225.   Information resources in toxicology, by Philip Wexler.
        New York: Elsevier/North-Holland, 1982.

226.   Information to authors, 1980-1981: editorial guidelines
        reproduced from 246 medical journals, by Harriett R.
        Meiss and Doris A. Jaeger. Baltimore: Urban &
        Schwarzenberg, 1980.

227.   Instructions for patients, by H. Winter Griffith. 3rd
        ed. Philadelphia: Saunders, 1982.

228.   Instrumentation for the operating room: a photographic
        manual, by Shirley M. Brooks. 2nd ed. St. Louis:
        Mosby, 1983.

229.   The International classification of diseases: 9th
        revision, clinical modification: ICD-9-CM. 2nd ed.
        Washington, DC: Health Care Financing Administration,
        1980. (3v.)

230.   International directory of specialized cancer research
        and treatment establishments. 3rd ed. Geneva:
        International Union Against Cancer, 1982.

231.   Interpretation of diagnostic tests: a handbook synopsis
        of laboratory medicine, by Jacques Wallach. 3rd ed.
        Boston: Little, Brown, 1978.

232.   Interpretation of pediatric tests, by Jacques Wallach.
        Boston: Little, Brown, 1983.

233.   Introduction to anesthesia: the principles of safe
        practice, by Robert Dunning Dripps, et al. 6th ed.
        Philadelphia: Saunders, 1982.

234.   Introduction to the history of medicine with medical
        chronology, suggestions for study and bibliographic
        data, by Fielding H. Garrison. 4th rev. and enl. ed.
        Philadelphia: Saunders, 1929.

235.   Inverted medical dictionary: a method of finding
        medical terms quickly, by Waldo A Rigal. Westport,
        CT: Technomic, 1976.

236.   Kidney, edited by Barry M. Brenner and Floyd C. Rector,
        Jr. 2nd ed. Philadelphia: Saunders, 1981. (2v.)

237. Krusen's handbook of physical medicine and rehabilita-
      tion, by Frederic J. Kottke, et al. 3rd ed. Phila-
      delphia: Saunders, 1982.

238. Labat's regional anesthesia: techniques and clinical
      applications, by John Adriani. 3rd ed. St. Louis:
      Warren H. Green, 1967.

239. Laboratory and diagnostic tests with nursing implica-
      tions, by Joyce LeFever Kee; with the assistance of
      Helen Liang Tang. Norwalk, CT: Appleton-Century-
      Crofts, 1983.

240. Laboratory medicine: hematology, by John B. Miale. 6th
      ed. St. Louis: Mosby, 1982.

241. Law every nurse should know, by Helen Creighton. 4th
      ed. Philadelphia: Saunders, 1981.

242. Lippincott manual of nursing practice, by Lillian
      Sholtis Brunner and Doris Smith Suddarth. 3rd ed.
      Philadelphia: Lippincott, 1982.

243. List of serials indexed for online users. Bethesda, MD:
      National Library of Medicine, 1980--. (annual)

244. MacBryde's signs and symptoms: applied pathologic
      physiology and clinical interpretation, by Robert S.
      Blacklow. 6th ed. Philadelphia: Lippincott, 1983.

245. McCance and Widdowson's the composition of foods, by A.
      A. Paul and D. A. T. Southgate. 4th ed. New York:
      Elsevier/North-Holland, 1978. (1980 supplement)

246. McGraw-Hill nursing dictionary. New York: McGraw-Hill,
      1979.

247. Major medicinal plants: botany, culture and uses, by
      Julia F. Morton. Springfield, IL: Thomas, 1977.

248. Major's physical diagnosis: an introduction to the
      clinical process, by Mahlon H. Delp and Robert T.
      Manning. 9th ed. Philadelphia: Saunders, 1981.

249. Manual for authors & editors: editorial style & manu-
      script preparation, compiled for the American Medical
      Association; edited by William R. Barclay, et al. 7th
      ed. Los Altos, CA: Lange, 1981.

250. Manual of clinical immunology, edited by Noel R. Rose
      and Herman Friedman. 2nd ed. Washington, DC:
      American Society for Microbiology, 1980.

251. Manual of clinical microbiology, edited by Edwin H.
      Lennette, et al. 3rd ed. Washington, DC: American
      Society for Microbiology, 1980.

252.   Manual of emergency pediatrics, edited by Robert M.
        Reece. 3rd ed. Philadelphia: Saunders, 1984.

253.   Manual of medical therapeutics, edited by J. William
        Campbell and Mark Frisse. 24th ed. Boston: Little,
        Brown, 1983.

254.   Manual of orthopaedic terminology, by Carolyn Talioferro
        Blauvelt and Fred R. T. Nelson. 2nd ed. St. Louis:
        Mosby, 1981.

255.   Manual of preoperative and postoperative care, by the
        Committee on Pre and Postoperative Care, American
        College of Surgeons. 3rd ed. Philadelphia:
        Saunders, 1983.

256.   Manual of skin diseases, by Gordon C. Sauer. 4th ed.
        Philadelphia: Lippincott, 1980.

257.   Martindale: the extra pharmacopoeia, edited by James E.
        F. Reynolds and Anne B. Prasad. 28th ed. London:
        Pharmaceutical Press, 1982.

258.   Maternity nursing, by Sharon J. Reeder, et al. 15th ed.
        Philadelphia: Lippincott, 1983.

259.   Maxcy-Rosenau public health and preventive medicine,
        edited by John M. Last. 11th ed. New York:
        Appleton-Century-Crofts, 1980.

260.   Medical abbreviations and acronyms, by Peter Roody, et
        al. New York: McGraw-Hill, 1977.

261.   Medical and health information directory, edited by
        Anthony T. Kruzas, et al. 2nd ed. Detroit: Gale,
        1980.

262.   Medical and health related sciences thesaurus.
        Bethesda, MD: National Institutes of Health, 1963--.
        (annual)

263.   Medical and healthcare marketplace guide, edited by
        Adeline B. Hale, et al. 3rd ed. Miami:
        International Bio-Medical Information Service, 1975--.
        (updated quarterly)

264.   A Medical bibliography (Garrison & Morton): an
        annotated check-list of texts illustrating the history
        of medicine, by Leslie T. Morton. 4th ed. Aldershot,
        Hampshire: Gower; Lexington, MA: distributed in the
        U.S. and Canada by Lexington Books, 1983.

265.   Medical books and serials in print. New York: Bowker,
        1978--.

266. Medical complications during pregnancy, edited by Gerard
     N. Burrow and Thomas F. Ferris. 2nd ed.
     Philadelphia: Saunders, 1982.

267. Medical device register: the official directory of
     hospital suppliers. Greenwich, CT: Directory
     Systems, 1981--. (annual)

268. Medical directory. London: Churchill Livingstone,
     1845--. (annual)

269. Medical embryology, by Jan Langman; original illustra-
     tions by Jill Leland. 4th ed. Baltimore: Williams &
     Wilkins, 1981.

270. Medical genetics: principles and practice, by James J.
     Nora and F. Clarke Fraser. 2nd ed. Philadelphia:
     Lea & Febiger, 1981.

271. Medical phrase index: a one-step reference to the termi-
     nology of medicine, edited by Jean A. Lorenzini.
     Oradell, NJ: Medical Economics, 1978.

272. Medical physiology, edited by Vernon B. Mountcastle.
     14th ed. St. Louis: Mosby, 1980.

273. Medical reference works, 1679-1966: a selected biblio-
     graphy, edited by John B. Blake and Charles Roos.
     Chicago: Medical Library Association, 1967. (supple-
     mented in 1970, 1973, and 1975)

274. Medical register. London: General Medical Council,
     1859--. (2v.)

275. Medical school admission requirements, United States and
     Canada. Washington, DC: Association of American
     Medical Colleges, 1978--. (annual)

276. Medical sign language: easily understood definitions of
     commonly used medical, dental and first aid terms, by
     W. Joseph Garcia. Springfield, IL: Thomas, 1983.

277. Medical-surgical nursing: concepts and clinical prac-
     tice, by Wilma J. Phipps, et al. 2nd ed. St. Louis:
     Mosby, 1983.

278. Medical terminology from Greek and Latin, by Sandra R.
     Patterson and Lawrence S. Thompson. Rev. ed. Troy,
     NY: Whitson, 1982.

279. Medical word finder, by George Willeford, Jr. 3rd ed.
     Englewood Cliffs, NJ: Prentice-Hall, 1983.

280. Medication teaching manual: a guide for patient
     counseling. 3rd ed. Bethesda, MD: American Society
     of Hospital Pharmacists, 1983.

281.   Medicine for the practicing physician, edited by J.
        Willis Hurst, et al. Boston: Butterworths, 1983.

282.   MEDOC: index to U.S. government publications in the
        medical and health sciences. Salt Lake City: Spencer
        S. Eccles Medical Sciences Library, University of
        Utah, 1968--. (quarterly with annual cumulation)

283.   Melloni's illustrated medical dictionary, by Ida Dox,
        et al. Baltimore: Williams & Wilkins, 1979.

284.   Mendelian inheritance in man: catalogs of autosomal
        dominant, autosomal recessive & x-linked phenotypes,
        by Victor A. McKusick. 6th ed. Baltimore: Johns
        Hopkins University Press, 1983.

285.   Merck index: an encyclopedia of chemicals, drugs, and
        biologicals, edited by Martha Windholz, et al. 10th
        ed. Rahway, NJ: Merck, 1983.

286.   Merck manual of diagnosis and therapy, edited by Robert
        Berkow, et al. 14th ed. Rahway, NJ: Merck, 1982.

287.   Metabolic basis of inherited disease, by John B. Stan-
        bury, et al. 5th ed. New York: McGraw-Hill, 1983.

288.   Metabolic control and disease, edited by Philip K. Bondy
        and Leon E. Rosenberg. 8th ed. Philadelphia:
        Saunders, 1980.

289.   Meyler's side effects of drugs, edited by Leopold Meyler
        and M. N. G. Dukes. New York: Elsevier/North-
        Holland, 1955--. (annual between editions: Side
        effects of drugs annual, edited by M. N. G. Dukes)

290.   MGH textbook of emergency medicine: emergency care as
        practiced at the Massachusetts General Hospital,
        edited by Earle W. Wilkins, et al. 2nd ed.
        Baltimore: Williams & Wilkins, 1983.

291.   Modern clinical psychiatry, by Lawrence C. Kolb and H.
        Keith Brodie. 10th ed. Philadelphia: Saunders,
        1982.

292.   Modern legal medicine, psychiatry, and forensic science,
        edited by William J. Curran, et al. Philadelphia:
        Davis, 1980.

293.   Modern nutrition in health and disease, edited by Robert
        S. Goodhart and Maurice E. Shils. 6th ed. Philadel-
        phia: Lea & Febiger, 1980.

294.   Mosby's manual of clinical nursing procedures, edited by
        Jane Hirsch and Leslie Hannock. St. Louis: Mosby,
        1981.

295. Mosby's manual of critical care, by Linda Feiwell Abels. St. Louis: Mosby, 1979.

296. Mosby's medical & nursing dictionary, edited by Laurence Urdang and Helen Harding Swallow. St. Louis: Mosby, 1983.

297. National directory of children & youth services: the reference handbook for professionals. Washington, DC: CPR Directory Services, 1979--. (annual)

298. National drug code directory. Rockville, MD: Food and Drug Administration, 1982. (quarterly supplements)

299. National health directory, edited by John T. Grupenhoff and Betty Farley. Rockville, MD: Aspen, 1977--. (annual)

300. National Library of Medicine audiovisuals catalog. Bethesda, MD: National Library of Medicine, 1977--. (quarterly with annual cumulation)

301. National Library of Medicine classification: a scheme for the shelf arrangement of books in the field of medicine and its related sciences. 4th rev. ed. Bethesda, MD: National Library of Medicine, 1981.

302. National Library of Medicine current catalog. Bethesda, MD: National Library of Medicine, 1966--. (quarterly with annual cumulation)

303. National nursing directory, edited by Kenneth E. Lawrence and Howard S. Rowland. Rockville, MD: Aspen, 1982.

304. Nelson textbook of pediatrics, by Richard E. Behrman and Victor C. Vaughan, III. 12th ed. Philadelphia: Saunders, 1983.

305. Neonatology: pathophysiology and management of the new-born, edited by Gordon G. Avery. 2nd ed. Philadel-phia: Lippincott, 1981.

306. Neurological surgery: a comprehensive reference guide to the diagnosis and management of neurosurgical problems, edited by Julian R. Youmans. 2nd ed. Philadelphia: Saunders, 1982. (6v.)

307. NIAID catalog of research reagents, edited by Sylvia Cunningham. Bethesda, MD: National Institute of Allergy and Infectious Diseases, 1977--. (triennial)

308. NLN nursing data book: statistical information on nursing education and newly licensed nurses. New York: National League for Nursing, 1978--. (annual)

309. Nomina anatomica: approved by the Eleventh
      International Congress of Anatomists at Mexico City,
      1980: together with Nomina histologica and Nomina
      embryologica; prepared by subcommittees of the
      International Anatomical Nomenclature Committee.
      Baltimore: Williams & Wilkins, 1983.

310. Novak's gynecologic and obstetric pathology with
      clinical and endocrine relations, by Edmund R. Novak
      and J. Donald Woodruff. 8th ed. Philadelphia:
      Saunders, 1979.

311. Novak's textbook of gynecology, by Howard W. Jones, Jr.
      and Georgeanna S. Jones. 10th ed. Baltimore:
      Williams & Wilkins, 1981.

312. Nurse's drug handbook, by Suzanne Loebl and George
      Spratto. 3rd ed. New York: Wiley, 1983.

313. Nurses' drug reference, by Joseph A. Albanese. 2nd ed.
      New York: McGraw-Hill, 1982. (1983 Update)

314. Nurses' handbook of fluid balance, by Norma Milligan
      Metheny and W. D. Snively, Jr. 4th ed. Philadelphia:
      Lippincott, 1983.

315. Nursing and allied health index. Glendale, CA: Glen-
      dale Adventist Medical Center, v. 22--, 1977--.
      (bimonthly with annual cumulation)

316. Nursing care in eye, ear, nose and throat disorders, by
      William H. Saunders, et al. 4th ed. St. Louis:
      Mosby, 1979.

317. Nursing Career Directory, by Eileen McGovern Cleary.
      Horsham, PA: Intermed Communications, 1979--. (annual)

318. Obstetrics and gynecology, edited by David N. Danforth,
      et al. 4th ed. Hagerstown, MD: Harper & Row, 1982.

319. Occupational diseases: a guide to their recognition,
      edited by Marcus M. Key. Rev. ed. Washington, DC:
      National Institute for Occupational Safety and Health,
      1977. (indexed by Index of signs and symptoms of
      industrial diseases)

320. Operative dentistry, by H. William Gilmore, et al. 4th
      ed. St. Louis: Mosby, 1982.

321. Operative obstetrics, by Edward J. Quilligan and
      Frederick Zuspan. 4th ed. New York: Appleton-
      Century-Crofts, 1982.

322. Ophthalmic surgery: principles and practice, edited by
      George L. Spaeth. Philadelphia: Saunders, 1982.

323. Ophthalmology: principles and concepts, by Frank W. Newell. 5th ed. St. Louis: Mosby, 1982.

324. Oral diagnosis, by Donald A. Kerr, et al. 6th ed. St. Louis: Mosby, 1983.

325. Origin of medical terms, by Henry Alan Skinner. 2nd ed., reprinted with corrections. New York: Hafner, 1970.

326. Orthopaedics: principles and their application, by Samuel L. Turek. 4th ed. Philadelphia: Lippincott, 1984. (2v.)

327. Orthopedic diseases: physiology, pathology, radiology, by Ernest Aegerter and John A. Kirkpatrick. 4th ed. Philadelphia: Saunders, 1975.

328. Otolaryngology, edited by Michael M. Paparella and Donald A. Shumrick. 2nd ed. Philadelphia: Saunders, 1980. (3v.)

329. Pathologic basis of disease, by Stanley L. Robbins, et al. 3rd ed. Philadelphia: Saunders, 1984.

330. Pathology, edited by W. A. D. Anderson and John M. Kissane. 7th ed. St. Louis: Mosby, 1977. (2v.)

331. Pathophysiology: the biological principles of disease, edited by Lloyd H. Smith, Jr. and Samuel O. Thier. Philadelphia: Saunders, 1981.

332. Patient care audit criteria: standards for hospital quality assurance, by Jean Gayton Carroll. 4th ed. Homewood, IL: Dow Jones-Irwin, 1983.

333. Patient care standards, by Susan Martin Tucker, et al. 3rd ed. St. Louis: Mosby, 1984.

334. Paul and Juhl's essentials of roentgen interpretation, by John H. Juhl. 4th ed. Hagerstown, MD: Harper & Row, 1981.

335. Pediatric clinical gastroenterology, by Arnold Silverman and Claude C. Roy. 3rd ed. St. Louis: Mosby, 1983.

336. Pediatric ophthalmology, edited by Robison D. Harley. 2nd ed. Philadelphia: Saunders, 1983. (2v.)

337. Pediatric orthopedics, by Mihran O. Tachdjian. Philadelphia: Saunders, 1972. (2v.)

338. Pediatric x-ray diagnosis: textbook for students and
      practitioners of pediatrics, surgery and radiology, by
      John Caffey, et al. 7th ed. Chicago: Year Book,
      1978. (2v.)

339. Pediatrics, edited by Abraham M. Rudolph, et al. 17th
      ed. Norwalk, CT: Appleton-Century-Crofts, 1982.

340. Periodical title abbreviations, edited by Leland G.
      Alkire, Jr. and Karen A. Olson. 4th ed. Detroit:
      Gale, 1983. (supplemented annually by New periodical
      title abbreviations) (3v.)

341. Peterson's annual guides to graduate study. Book 3,
      Biological, agricultural, and health sciences, edited
      by Karen C. Hegener. Princeton, NJ: Peterson's
      Guides, 1976--. (annual)

342. Pharmacological and chemical synonyms: a collection of
      names of drugs, pesticides and other compounds drawn
      from the medical literature of the world, by E. E. J.
      Marler. 7th ed. New York: Elsevier/North-Holland,
      1983.

343. Pharmacology and pharmacologists: an international
      directory. New York: Oxford University Press, 1981.

344. PharmIndex: professional product information for
      pharmacists. Portland, OR: Skyline Publishers,
      1958--. (loose-leaf) (monthly)

345. Physical evaluation of the dental patient, by Charles L.
      Halstead, et al. St. Louis: Mosby, 1982.

346. Physician characteristics and distribution in the U.S.
      Chicago: American Medical Association, 1982--.
      (annual)

347. Physicians' current procedural terminology, by Steven B.
      Clauser, et al. 4th rev. ed. Chicago: American
      Medical Association, 1983.

348. Physicians' desk reference. Oradell, NJ: Medical
      Economics, 1974--. (annual)

349. Physicians' desk reference for nonprescription drugs.
      Oradell, NJ: Medical Economics, 1980--. (annual)

350. Physician's handbook, by Marcus A. Krupp, et al. 20th
      ed. Los Altos, CA: Lange, 1982.

351. Poisoning: toxicology--symptoms--treatments, by Jay M.
      Arena. 4th ed. Springfield, IL: Thomas, 1979.

352. Poisonous and venomous marine animals of the world, by
     Bruce W. Halstead; with editorial assistance of Linda
     G. Halstead. Rev. ed. Princeton, NJ: Darwin, 1978.

353. Poisonous plants of the United States and Canada, by
     John M. Kingsbury. Englewood Cliffs, NJ: Prentice-
     Hall, 1964.

354. A Practical approach to infectious diseases, edited by
     Richard E. Reese and R. Gordon Douglas, Jr. Boston:
     Little, Brown, 1983.

355. Principles and practice of infectious diseases, edited
     by Gerald L. Mandell, et al. New York: Wiley, 1979.
     (2v.)

356. Principles and practice of medicine, edited by A.
     McGehee Harvey, et al. 21st ed. New York: Appleton-
     Century-Crofts, 1984.

357. Principles and techniques in pediatric nursing, by
     Gloria Leifer. 4th ed. Philadelphia: Saunders,
     1982.

358. Principles of ambulatory medicine, edited by L. Randol
     Barker, et al. Baltimore: Williams & Wilkins, 1982.

359. Principles of neurology, by Raymond D. Adams and Maurice
     Victor. 2nd ed. New York: McGraw-Hill, 1981.

360. Principles of surgery, edited by Seymour I. Schwartz, et
     al. 4th ed. New York: McGraw-Hill, 1984.

361. Proceedings in print. Arlington, MA: Proceedings in
     Print, 1964--. (bimonthly with annual cumulation)

362. Professional resume and job search guide, by Harold W.
     Dickhut. 5th ed. Englewood Cliffs, NJ: Prentice-
     Hall, 1981.

363. Profile of medical practice. Chicago: American Medical
     Association, 1978--. (annual)

364. Psychiatric dictionary, by Robert Jean Campbell. 5th
     ed. New York: Oxford University Press, 1981.

365. Pulmonary diseases and disorders, edited by Alfred P.
     Fishman. New York: McGraw-Hill, 1980. (2v.) (1982
     Update)

366. Pulmonary medicine, edited by Clarence A. Guenter and
     Martin H. Welch. 2nd ed. Philadelphia: Lippincott,
     1982.

367. Radiology of emergency medicine, by John H. Harris, Jr.
      and William H. Harris. 2nd ed. Baltimore: Williams
      & Wilkins, 1981.

368. Radiology of syndromes and metabolic disorders, by
      Hooshang Taybi. 2nd ed. Chicago: Year Book, 1983.

369. Reconstructive plastic surgery: principles, procedures
      in correction, reconstruction and transplantation,
      edited by John Marquis Converse, et al. 2nd ed.
      Philadelphia: Saunders, 1977. (7v.)

370. Registry of toxic effects of chemical substances.
      Cincinnati: National Institute for Occupational
      Safety and Health, 1975--. (annual)

371. Remington's pharmaceutical sciences, edited by Arthur
      Osol. 16th ed. Easton, PA: Mack, 1980.

372. Renal and electrolyte disorders, edited by Robert W.
      Schrier. 2nd ed. Boston: Little, Brown, 1980.

373. Report of the Committee on Infectious Diseases, American
      Academy of Pediatrics. 19th ed. Evanston, IL: The
      Academy, 1982.

374. Research awards index. Bethesda, MD: National Insti-
      tutes of Health, Division of Research Grants, 16th
      ed.--, 1976--. (annual)

375. Research centers directory: a guide to university-
      related and other nonprofit organizations, edited by
      Mary Michelle Watkins and James A. Ruffner. 8th ed.
      Detroit: Gale, 1983. (supplemented quarterly by New
      research centers)

376. Research programs in the medical sciences, edited by
      Jaques Cattell Press. New York: Bowker, 1981--.
      (biennial)

377. Reversicon: a medical word finder, by J. E. Schmidt.
      Springfield, IL: Thomas, 1958.

378. Review of medical physiology, by William F. Ganong.
      Los Altos, CA: Lange, 1963--. (biennial)

379. Rob & Smith's operative surgery, series edited by
      Charles Rob and Rodney Smith. 4th ed. Boston:
      Butterworths, 1983--.

380. Rypins' medical licensure examinations: topical
      summaries and questions, edited by Edward D. Frohlich.
      13th ed. Philadelphia: Lippincott, 1981.

381. Saunders health care directory 84/85. Philadelphia:
      Saunders, 1984.

382. Schaffer's diseases of the newborn, by Mary Ellen Avery
      and H. William Taeusch, Jr. 5th ed. Phialdelphia:
      Saunders, 1984.

383. Science citation index. Philadelphia: Institute for
      Scientific Information, 1961--. (bimonthly with
      annual cumulation)

384. Scientific American medicine, edited by Edward
      Rubenstein and Daniel D. Federman. New York:
      Scientific American, 1978--. (loose-leaf) (monthly)

385. Scientific, engineering, and medical societies
      publications in print. New York: Bowker, 1977--.
      (biennial)

386. Scientific meetings. San Diego: Scientific Meetings
      Publications, 1957--. (quarterly)

387. Smith's reference and illustrated guide to surgical
      instruments, by E. J. Smith and Y. R. Smith. Phila-
      delphia: Lippincott, 1983.

388. Sodeman's pathologic physiology: mechanisms of disease,
      edited by William A. Sodeman, Jr. and William A.
      Sodeman. 6th ed. Philadelphia: Saunders, 1979.

389. Sourcebook on death and dying, edited by James A.
      Fruehling. Chicago: Marquis Professional Publica-
      tions, 1982.

390. Statistical abstract of the United States. Washington,
      DC: Bureau of the Census, 1878--. (annual)

391. Stedman's medical dictionary. 24th ed. Baltimore:
      Williams & Wilkins, 1982.

392. Strauss and Welt's diseases of the kidney, edited by
      Lawrence E. Earley and Carl W. Gottschalk. 3rd ed.
      Boston: Little, Brown, 1979. (2v.)

393. Surgery of the alimentary tract, by Richard T.
      Shackelford and George D. Zuidema. 2nd ed. Philadel-
      phia: Saunders, 1978--.

394. Surgery of the anus, rectum and colon, by John C.
      Goligher. 5th ed. Philadelphia: Saunders, 1984.

395. Surgical infectious diseases, edited by Richard L.
      Simmons and Richard J. Howard. New York: Appleton-
      Century-Crofts, 1982.

396. Surgical radiology: a complement in radiology and
      imaging to the Sabiston Davis-Christopher textbook of
      surgery, edited by J. George Teplick and Marvin E.
      Haskin. Philadelphia: Saunders, 1981. (3v.)

397. Swenson's pediatric surgery, by John G. Raffensperger.
      4th ed. Norwalk, CT: Appleton-Century-Crofts, 1980.

398. Systematized nomenclature of medicine, edited by Roger
      A. Cote. 2nd ed. Skokie, IL: College of American
      Pathologists, 1979. (1982 supplement)

399. Systemic disease in dental treatment, by Michael J.
      Tullman and Spencer W. Redding. New York: Appleton-
      Century-Crofts, 1982.

400. Taber's cyclopedic medical dictionary, edited by Clayton
      L. Thomas. 14th ed. Philadelphia: Davis, 1981.

401. Te Linde's operative gynecology, by Richard F.
      Mattingly. 5th ed. Philadelpha: Lippincott, 1977.

402. Textbook of anatomy & physiology, by Catherine Parker
      Anthony and Gary A. Thibodeau; illustrated by Ernest
      W. Beck. 11th ed. St. Louis: Mosby, 1983.

403. Textbook of biochemistry with clinical correlations,
      edited by Thomas M. Devlin. New York: Wiley, 1982.

404. Textbook of diagnostic ultrasonography, by Sandra L.
      Hagen-Ansert. 2nd ed. St. Louis: Mosby, 1983.

405. Textbook of endocrinology, edited by Robert H. Williams.
      6th ed. Philadelphia: Saunders, 1981.

406. Textbook of family practice, edited by Robert E. Rakel.
      3rd ed. Philadelphia: Saunders, 1984.

407. Textbook of medical physiology, by Arthur C. Guyton.
      6th ed. Philadelphia: Saunders, 1981.

408. Textbook of neurology, edited by Lewis P. Rowland. 7th
      ed. Philadelphia: Lea & Febiger, 1984.

409. Textbook of oral and maxillofacial surgery, edited by
      Gustav O. Kruger. 6th ed. St. Louis: Mosby, 1984.

410. Textbook of oral pathology, by William G. Shafer, et al.
      4th ed. Philadelphia: Saunders, 1983.

411. Textbook of otolaryngology, by David D. DeWeese and
      William H. Saunders. 6th ed. St. Louis: Mosby,
      1982.

412. Textbook of pediatric emergency medicine, edited by Gary
      Fleisher and Steven Ludwig. Baltimore: Williams &
      Wilkins, 1983.

413. Textbook of pulmonary diseases, edited by Gerald L. Baum
      and Emanuel Wolinsky. 3rd ed. Boston: Little,
      Brown, 1983.

414.   Textbook of rheumatology, edited by William N. Kelley,
       et al. Philadelphia: Saunders, 1981.

415.   Textbook of surgery: the biological basis of modern
       surgical practice, edited by David C. Sabiston, Jr.
       12th ed. Philadelphia: Saunders, 1981.

416.   Textbook of veterinary internal medicine: diseases of
       the dog and cat, edited by Stephen J. Ettinger.   2nd
       ed. Philadelphia: Saunders, 1983. (2v.)

417.   Thoracic and cardiovascular surgery, edited by William
       W. L. Glenn, et al. 4th ed. Norwalk, CT: Appleton-
       Century-Crofts, 1983.

418.   Todd, Sanford, Davidsohn clinical diagnosis and manage-
       ment by laboratory methods, edited by John Bernard
       Henry. 17th ed. Philadelphia: Saunders, 1984.

419.   Treatment of injuries to athletes, by Don H. O'Donoghue.
       4th ed. Philadelphia: Saunders, 1984.

420.   Ulrich's international periodicals directory. New York:
       Bowker, 1932--.

421.   Understanding medical terminology, by Agnes Clare
       Frenay; illustrated by Helen M. Smith. 6th ed.   St.
       Louis: Catholic Hospital Association, 1977.

422.   Unlisted drugs. New York: Special Libraries Associa-
       tion, 1949--. (monthly)

423.   U.S. government manual. Washington, DC: Office of
       Federal Register, 1935--. (annual)

424.   U.S. medical directory. 6th ed. Miami: U.S. Directory
       Service, 1983.

425.   U.S. medical licensure statistics and licensure require-
       ments. Chicago: American Medical Association,
       1982--.

426.   U.S. pharmacopeia (20th ed.) & National formulary (15th
       ed.). Rockville, MD: United States Pharmacopeial
       Convention, 1979.

427.   U.S. pharmacopeia dispensing information: advice for
       the patient. Rockville, MD: United States
       Pharmacopeial Convention, 1983--. (v. 2) (annual)

428.   U.S. pharmacopeia dispensing information for the health
       care provider. Rockville, MD: United States Pharma-
       copeial Convention, 1983--. (v. 1) (annual)

429.   USAN and the USP dictionary of drug names, edited by
       Mary C. Griffiths, et al. Rockville, MD: United
       States Pharmacopeial Convention, 1971--. (annual)

430.   Vaccination certificate requirements for international
       travellers. Geneva: World Health Organization,
       1981--. (annual)

431.   Vascular surgery, edited by Robert B. Rutherford. 2nd
       ed. Philadelphia: Saunders, 1984.

432.   Veterinary medicine: a textbook of the diseases of
       cattle, sheep, pigs, goats and horses, by D. C. Blood,
       et al. 6th ed. London: Bailliere Tindall, 1983.

433.   Veterinary pathology, by Thomas Carlyle Jones and Ronald
       Duncan Hunt. 5th ed. Philadelphia: Lea & Febiger,
       1983.

434.   Veterinary pharmaceuticals & biologicals, edited by Carl
       E. Aronson. Media, PA: Harwal, 1981--. (biennial)

435.   Veterinary pharmacology and therapeutics, edited by
       Nicholas H. Booth and Leslie E. McDonald. 5th ed.
       Ames: Iowa State University, 1982.

436.   Vital and health statistics series. Hyattsville, MD:
       National Center for Health Statistics, 1963--.

437.   Vital statistics of the United States. Washington, DC:
       National Center for Health Statistics, 1937--.
       (annual) (3v.)

438.   Whole nurse catalog, by Jane Jackson. Philadelphia:
       Saunders, 1980.

439.   Whole pediatrician catalog: a compendium of clues to
       diagnosis and management, by Julia A. McMillan, et al.
       Philadelphia: Saunders, 1977--.

440.   Who's who in health care. 2nd ed. New York: Hanover,
       1981.

441.   Williams obstetrics, by Jack A. Pritchard and Paul C.
       MacDonald. 16th ed. New York: Appleton-Century-
       Crofts, 1980.

442.   World directory of medical schools. 5th ed. Geneva:
       World Health Organization, 1979.

443.   World health statistics annual. Geneva: World Health
       Organization, 1962--. (3v.)

444.   World meetings: medicine. New York: Macmillan,
       1978--. (quarterly)

445. World of learning. London: Europa; Detroit: distrib-
      uted by Gale, 1947--. (annual)

446. Yearbook of international organizations. Brussels:
      Union of International Associations, 1949--.

447. Young's learning medical terminology step by step:
      textbook and workbook, by Miriam G. Austrin.   5th ed.
      St. Louis: Mosby, 1983.

ALTERNATE TITLE INDEX

AHA guide to the health care field 184

American Medical Association directory of officials and staff 14

American Medical Association drug evaluations 15

Atlas of anatomy 180

Care of the patient in surgery 11

Ciba-Geigy scientific tables 170

CINAHL 315

Clinical diagnosis and management by laboratory methods 418

Clinical laboratory methods and diagnosis 179

Composite index for CRC handbooks 93

Composition of foods 245

Computerized index to U.S. government documents in the medical and health sciences 282

Conn's current therapy 111

CPT 347

Craig and Faust's clinical parasitology 83

Cumulated index medicus 218

Cumulative index to nursing & allied health literature 315

Current catalog 302

Current drug handbook 160

Current procedural terminology 347

CVP 113

Cyclopedic medical dictionary 400

Davis-Christopher textbook of surgery 415

Diagnostic microbiology 35

Dictionary of biological terms 209

Directory of accredited residencies 128

Diseases of the kidney 392

Diseases of the newborn 382

Diseases of the skin 26

Douglas-Stromme operative obstetrics 321

Drug code directory 298

Drug facts and comparisons 158

DSM-III 118

Essentials of roentgen interpretation 334

Extra pharmacopoeia 257

Family medical guide 21

Food values of portions commonly used 54

Gould medical dictionary 52

Gray's anatomy of the human body 25

Gynecologic and obstetric pathology 310

Handbook of biochemistry and molecular biology 94

Handbook of chemistry and
  physics 95
Handbook of engineering in
  medicine and biology 96
Handbook of laboratory
  animal science 97
Handbook of microbiology 98
Handbook of physical medicine
  and rehabilitation 237
Handbook series in clinical
  laboratory science 99
Illustrated medical
  dictionary 283
Index of differential
  diagnosis 166
Index of signs and symptoms
  of industrial diseases 319
Index to U.S. government
  publications in the medical
  and health sciences 282
Internship and residency
  announcements 178
Learning medical terminology
  step by step 447
Management of fractures and
  dislocations 115
Manual of determinative
  bacteriology 39
Massachusetts General
  Hospital textbook of
  emergency medicine 290
Merritt's textbook of
  neurology 408
MeSH thesaurus 262
Neurological and
  neurosurgical nursing 63
NLM audiovisuals catalog 300
NLM current catalog 302
Nursing data book 308
Occupational diseases 220

Operative gynecology 401
Operative orthopedics 56
Operative surgery 379
Pathologic physiology 388
PDR 348
PDR for nonprescription drugs
  349
Pharmacological basis of
  therapeutics 175
Physical diagnosis 248
Physiological basis of medical
  practice 40
Public health and preventive
  medicine 259
Red book 373
Reece-Chamberlain manual of
  emergency pediatrics 252
Reference and illustrated
  guide to surgical
  instruments 387
RTECS 370
Scientific tables 170
Side effects of drugs 289
Signs and symptoms 244
SNOMED 398
Surgery of the chest 173
Surgical pathology 8
Textbook of emergency medicine
  290
Textbook of gynecology 311
Textbook of medicine 67
Textbook of neurology 408
Textbook of pediatrics 304
Tropical medicine 215
United States adopted names
  423
United States statistical
  abstract 390
USP DI 427, 428
VPB 434

AUTHOR INDEX

Abels, Linda Feiwell 295
Adams, Raymond D. 359
Adriani, John 238
Aegerter, Ernest 327
Albanese, Joseph A. 313
Alexander, Edythe Louise 11
Alkire, Leland G., Jr. 340
Altman, Norman H. 97
Altman, Philip L. 48
Alvarado, Don M. 25
American Academy of
  Pediatrics 373
American Association for the
  Advancement of Science
  183
American Association of
  Dental Schools 10
American Board of Medical
  Specialties 126
American Cancer Society 59
American College of Hospital
  Administrators 123
American College of
  Physicians 45
American College of Surgeons
  16, 255
American Dental Association
  5, 17
American Dietetic Association
  187
American Geriatrics Society
  72
American Hospital Association
  184, 211, 212

American Library Association
  182
American Medical Association
  13, 14, 15, 21, 22, 128,
  130, 249, 346, 347, 363,
  425
American Nurses' Association
  157
American Pharmaceutical
  Association 156, 190
American Psychiatric
  Association 44, 118
American Public Health
  Association 46, 91
American Society for
  Microbiology 250, 251
American Society of Hospital
  Pharmacists 20, 194, 280
American Type Culture
  Collection 65, 66
Anderson, James E. 180
Anderson, W. A. D. 330
Andrews, George C. 26
Anthony, Catherine Parker 402
Arena, Jay M. 351
Aronson, Carl E. 434
Association of American
  Medical Colleges 1, 2, 275
Association of Community
  Cancer Centers 86
Austrin, Miriam G. 447
Avery, Gordon G. 305
Avery, Mary Ellen 382
Bailey, W. Robert 35
Baker, A. B. 82

Baker, L. H.   82
Barber, Janet M.   144
Barclay, William R.   249
Barker, L. Randol   358
Bates, Barbara   181
Baum, Gerald L.   413
Beaver, Paul Chester   83
Beck, Ernest W.   402
Behrman, Richard E.   304
Benenson, Abram S.   91
Benson, Ralph C.   106, 191
Bergsma, Daniel   49
Berkow, Robert   286
Bernstein, Jerrold G.   189
Best, Charles H.   40
Biller, Jeffrey A.   195
Billups, Norman F.   18
Billups, Shirley M.   18
Blacklow, Robert S.   244
Blake, John B.   273
Blauvelt, Carolyn Talioferro
   254
Blood, D. C.   432
Bockus, Henry L.   168
Boever, William J.   131
Bondy, Philip K.   288
Booth, Nicholas H.   435
Borgaonkar, Digamber S.   69
Boucher, Carl O.   101
Bowes, Anna de Planter   54
Braunwald, Eugene   206
Brenner, Barry M.   236
Briggs, William E.   178
Brodie, H. Keith   291
Brooks, Shirley M.   228
Brunner, Lillian Sholtis   242
Buchanan, R. E.   39
Buchsbaum, Herbert J.   185
Budassi, Susan A.   144
Bureau of the Census   390
Burrow, Gerard N.   266
Buschle, Kay Brown   167
Caffey, John   338
Campbell, J. William   253
Campbell, Meredith F.   57
Campbell, Robert Jean   364
Campbell, Willis C.   56
Canadian Hospital Association
   58
Carini, Esta   63
Carroll, Jean Gayton   332
Catholic Hospital Association
   421
Cecil, Russell L.   67
Chatton, Milton J.   105
Chen, Ching-chih   201

Christopher, Frederick   415
Church, Helen Nichols   54
Chusid, Joseph G.   92
Clark, Mary Virginia   273
Clauser, Steven B.   347
Cleary, Eileen McGovern   317
College of American
   Pathologists   398
Conn, Howard F.   104, 111
Conn, Rex B.   104
Connolly, John F.   115
Converse, John Marquis   369
Conway-Rutkowski, Barbara Lang
   63
Cote, Roger A.   398
Cotran, Ramzi S.   329
Crawford, Susan   125
Creighton, Helen   241
Crenshaw, A. H.   56
Crowley, Ellen T.   9
Cunningham, Sylvia   307
Curran, William J.   292
Danforth, David N.   318
Darnay, Brigitte T.   129
Daun, Lowell G.   210
Davidsohn, Israel   418
Davis, Loyal E.   415
DeGowin, Elmer L.   38
DeGowin, Richard L.   38
DeGroot, Leslie J.   153
Delp, Mahlon H.   248
del Regato, Juan A.   7
De Palma, Anthony F.   115
DeVita, Vincent T.   61
Devlin, Thomas M.   403
DeWeese, David D.   411
Dickhut, Harold W.   362
Dittmer, Dorothy S.   48
Domonkos, Anthony N.   26
Dorland, W. A. Newman   134
Douglas, R. Gordon   321, 354
Dox, Ida   283
Dreisbach, Robert H.   193
Dripps, Robert Dunning   233
Dukes, M. N. G.   289
Earley, Lawrence E.   392
Edmonson, Allen S.   56
Ethridge, J. M.   124
Ettinger, Stephen J.   416
Farley, Betty   299
Fasman, Gerald D.   94
Federation of American
   Societies for Experimental
   Biology   48
Federman, Daniel D.   384
Feigenbaum, Harvey   140

Feinberg, Barry N.   96
Ferris, Thomas F.   266
Finegold, Sydney M.   35
Fiore, Mariano S. H. di   33
Fishman, Alfred P.   365
Fitzpatrick, Thomas B.   116
Fleisher, Gary   412
Fleming, David G.   96
Food and Drug Administration
   298
Fordtran, John S.   169
Foundation Center   163, 164
Fraser, F. Clarke   270
Fraser, Robert G.   117
Frei, Emil   60
Frenay, Agnes Clare   421
French, Herbert   166
Friedman, Herman   250
Frisse, Mark   253
Frohlich, Edward D.   380
Fruehling, James A.   389
Ganong, William F.   378
Garcia, W. Joseph   276
Garrison, Fielding H.   234,
   264
Gellis, Sydney S.   109
Gennaro, Alfonso R.   52
Gibbon, John H.   173
Gibbons, N. E.   39
Gilman, Alfred Goodman   175
Gilmore, H. William   320
Glendale Adventist Medical
   Center   315
Glenn, William W. L.   417
Goligher, John C.   394
Goodhart, Robert S.   293
Goss, Charles Mayo   25
Gosselin, Robert E.   85
Gottschalk, Carl W.   392
Gourman, Jack   176, 177
Govoni, Laura E.   137
Gradwohl, R. B. H.   179
Grant, J. C. Boileau   180
Gray, Henry   25
Green, David P.   165
Greenspan, Ezra M.   79
Griffith, H. Winter   227
Griffiths, Mary C.   423
Gruendemann, Barbara J.   11
Grupenhoff, John T.   299
Guenter, Clarence A.   366
Guyton, Arthur C.   407
Hagen-Ansert, Sandra L.   404
Hale, Adeline B.   263
Halstead, Bruce W.   352
Halstead, Charles L.   345

Halstead, Linda G.   352
Hannock, Leslie   294
Hansten, Philip D.   135
Harley, Robison D.   336
Harris, John H., Jr.   367
Harris, William H.   367
Harrison, J. Hartwell   57
Hart, F. Dudley   166
Harvey, A. McGehee   122, 356
Haskin, Marvin E.   396
Hayes, Janice E.   137
Health Care Financing
   Administration   229
Hegener, Karen C.   341
Henderson, Isabella F.   209
Henning, Margaret   125
Henry, John Bernard   418
Hirsch, Jane   294
Hoeprich, Paul D.   223
Holland, James F.   60
Hollinshead, W. Henry   24
Holmes, Sandra   209
Hooley, James R.   210
Howard, Richard J.   395
Hudak, Carolyn M.   100
Huffman, John W.   186
Hughes, Harold K.   119
Hunt, Ronald Duncan   433
Hunter, George W.   215
Hurst, J. Willis   205, 281
Huth, Edward J.   213
Institute for Scientific,
   Information   102, 103, 221,
   222
International Anatomical
   Nomenclature Committee   309
International Union Against
   Cancer   230
Jablonski, Stanley   216, 217
Jackson, Jane   438
Jaeger, Doris A.   226
Jarett, Leonard   179
Johns Hopkins University   195
Joint Commission on
   Accreditation of Hospitals
   6
Jones, Georgeanna S.   311
Jones, Howard W., Jr.   311
Jones, Thomas Carlyle   433
Juhl, John H.   334
Kagan, Benjamin M.   109
Kaplan, Harold I.   89
Kaplan, Norman M.   78
Kaszubski, Marek   198
Katcher, Brian S.   30
Katz, Jordan   28

Katz, Samuel L. 224
Kaufman, Joseph J. 112
Keane, Claire Brackman 145
Keckeissen, Rita G. 182
Kee, Joyce LeFever 239
Kelley, William N. 414
Kelly, Emerson Crosby 152
Kempe, C. Henry 108
Kerr, Donald A. 324
Kingsbury, John M. 353
Kirk, R. W. 113
Kirkpatrick, John A. 327
Kissane, John M. 330
Kleeman, Charles R. 74
Knoben, James E. 188
Kolb, Lawrence C. 291
Kottke, Frederic J. 237
Kravis, Thomas Clarke 142
Kruger, Gustav O. 409
Krugman, Saul 224
Krupp, Marcus A. 105, 350
Krusen, Frank H. 237
Kruzas, Anthony T. 151, 203,
  261
Kunz, Jeffrey R. M. 21
Lachmann, P. J. 73
Langman, Jan 269
Laskin, Allen I. 98
Last, John M. 259
Lawrence, Kenneth E. 303
Lechevalier, Hubert A. 98
Lehninger, Albert L. 43
Leifer, Gloria 357
Leiter, Elliot 107
Lennette, Edwin H. 251
Lentner, C. 170
Leung, Albert Y. 149
Loebl, Suzanne 312
Lore, John M. 32
Lorenzini, Jean A. 271
Ludwig, Steven 412
McCarthy, Daniel J. 31
McDonald, Leslie E. 435
MacDonald, Paul C. 441
McIlvaine, Eileen 182
McKusick, Victor A. 284
McMillan, Julia A. 439
Magalini, Sergio I. 121
Maingot, Rodney 4
Major, Ralph H. 71, 248
Mandell, Gerald L. 355
Manning, Robert T. 248
Marler, E. E. J. 342
Marlow, C. A. 124
Martin, William J. 35

Massachusetts General Hospital
  290
Mattingly, Richard F. 401
Maxcy, Kenneth Fuller 259
Maxwell, Morton H. 74
Medical Economics 348, 349
Medical Library Association
  273
Meeker, Margaret Huth 11
Meiss, Harriett R. 226
Melby, Edward C. 97
Merritt, H. Houston 408
Metheny, Norma Milligan 314
Metzger, Norman 197
Meyler, Leopold 289
Miale, John B. 240
Middleton, Elliott, Jr. 12
Miller, Benjamin F. 145
Miller, Ronald D. 27
Modell, Walter 138, 139
Morton, Julia F. 247
Morton, Leslie T. 264
Moskowitz, Roland W. 84
Mountcastle, Vernon B. 272
Narrow, Barbara W. 167
Nathan, David G. 208
National Center for Health
  Statistics 159, 199, 204,
  436, 437
National Institute for
  Occupational Safety and
  Health 220, 319, 370
National Institute of Allergy
  and Infectious Diseases 307
National Institutes of Health
  87, 262
National League for Nursing
  308
National Library of Medicine
  42, 202, 218, 219, 243, 300,
  301, 302
Nelson, Fred R. T. 254
Nelson, Waldo Emerson 304
Netter, Frank H. 70
Newell, Frank W. 323
Nora, James J. 270
Novak, Edmund R. 310, 311
O'Donoghue, Don H. 419
Office of Federal Register
  423
Olson, Karen A. 340
Oski, Frank A. 208
Osol, Arthur 371
Owens, Guy 63
Paparella, Michael M. 328
Pare, J. A. Peter 117

Patterson, Sandra R.   278
Paul, A. A.   245
Paul, Lester W.   334
Pennington, Jean A. T.   54
Peters, D. K.   73
Petersdorf, Robert G.   196
Phipps, Wilma J.   277
Prasad, Anne B.   257
Pritchard, Jack A.   441
Quilligan, Edward J.   321
Raffensperger, John G.   397
Rakel, Robert E.   111, 406
Rector, Floyd C., Jr.   236
Redding, Spencer W.   399
Reece, Robert M.   252
Reeder, Sharon J.   258
Rees, Alan M.   90, 125
Reese, Richard E.   354
Reich, Warren T.   148
Reichel, William   72
Remington, Joseph P.   371
Renz, Loren   163
Reynolds, James E. F.   257
Richmond, Joy S.   273
Rigal, Waldo A.   235
Rob, Charles   379
Robbins, Laurence L.   174
Robbins, Stanley L.   329
Rockwood, Charles A., Jr.
  165
Roody, Peter   260
Roos, Charles   273
Rosai, Juan   8
Rose, Noel R.   250
Rosen, Peter   143
Rosenau, M. J.   259
Rosenberg, Leon E.   288
Rowland, Howard S.   303
Roy, Claude C.   335
Rubenstein, Edward   384
Rudolph, Abraham M.   339
Ruffner, James A.   375
Rutherford, Robert B.   431
Rypins, Harold D.   380
Sabiston, David C., Jr.
  173, 415
Sanford, Arthur H.   418
Sauer, Gordon C.   256
Saunders, William H.   316,
  411
Sax, N. Irving   114
Schiff, Eugene R.   132
Schiff, Leon   132
Schmidt, J. E.   377
Schmidt, Joseph D.   185
Schmittroth, John, Jr.   150

Schrier, Robert W.   372
Schwartz, Seymour I.   360
Schweer, Kathryn D.   34
Scipien, Gladys M.   88
Scott, Elvyn G.   35
Scrascia, Euclide   121
Seligson, David   99
Shackelford, Richard T.   393
Shafer, William G.   410
Shearer, Barbara S.   162
Shearer, Benjamin F.   162
Sheehy, Eugene P.   182
Shepard, Thomas H.   64
Sheridan, Eleanor   160
Sherlock, Sheila   133
Shils, Maurice E.   293
Shumrick, Donald A.   328
Silver, Henry K.   192
Silverman, Arnold   335
Simmons, Richard L.   395
Skinner, Henry Alan   325
Sleisenger, Marvin H.   169
Sliosberg, A.   141
Smith, Donald R.   172
Smith, E. J.   387
Smith, Helen M.   421
Smith, Lloyd H., Jr.   67, 331
Smith, Robert M.   29
Smith, Rodney   379
Smith, Y. R.   387
Snively, W. D., Jr.   314
Sodeman, William A.   388
Sodeman, William A., Jr.   388
Sonnenwirth, Alex C.   179
Southgate, D. A. T.   245
Spaeth, George L.   322
Special Libraries Association
  422
Spencer, Frank C.   173
Speroff, Leon   76
Spiro, Howard M.   75
Spittell, John A.   81
Spjut, Harlan J.   7
Spratto, George   312
Stanbury, John B.   287
Stanton, Sharon L.   129
Stedman, Thomas Lathrop   391
Steen, Edwin B.   3
Stites, Daniel P.   37
Strauss, Maurice B.   161
Strickland, G. Thomas   215
Stromme, William B.   321
Suddarth, Doris Smith   242
Swallow, Helen Harding   296
Taber, Clarence W.   400
Tachdjian, Mihran O.   337

Taeusch, H. William, Jr.   382
Talbott, John H.   47
Tang, Helen Liang   239
Taybi, Hooshang   368
Taylor, Norman B.   40
Te Linde, Richard W.   401
Teplick, J. George   396
Thibodeau, Gary A.   402
Thier, Samuel O.   331
Thomas, Clayton L.   400
Thompson, Lawrence S.   278
Thomson, William A. R.   50
Timmreck, Thomas   120
Todd, James C.   418
Trissel, Lawrence A.   194
Tucker, Susan Martin   333
Tullman, Michael J.   399
Turek, Samuel L.   326
Underhill, Sandra L.   62
Union of International
   Associations   446
United States Pharmacopeial
   Convention   426, 427, 428,
   429
Urdang, Lawrence   296
Vaughan, Daniel   171
Vaughan, Victor C., III   304
Victor, Maurice   359
Wallach, Jacques   231, 232
Wallach, Joel D.   131
Warner, Carmen Germaine   142
Warner, Steven D.   34

Washington University,
   St. Louis   253
Wasserman, Paul   198
Watkins, Mary Michelle   375
Way, Lawrence W.   110
Welch, Martin H.   366
West, Geoffrey P.   51, 146
West, John B.   40
Wexler, Philip   225
Whitehead, E. Douglas   107
Widdowson, E. M.   245
Widmann, Frances K.   80
Wilkins, Earle W.   290
Willeford, George, Jr.   279
Williams, Robert H.   405
Williams, William J.   207
Windholz, Martha   285
Wintrobe, Maxwell M.   77
Wischnitzer, Saul   36
Wolinsky, Emanuel   413
Woodruff, J. Donald   310
Woods, Nancy Fugate   214
World Health Organization
   430, 442, 443
Wyngaarden, James   67
Yeager, Andrew M.   195
Youmans, Julian R.   306
Young, Blanche A.   90
Young, Clara Gene   447
Zuidema, George D.   393
Zuspan, Frederick   321

THESAURUS-INDEX

ABBREVIATIONS

    RT   Acronyms
    RT   Initialisms
     Allied health sciences
      260
     Biochemistry   9, 43
     Biology   209
     Dentistry   3, 216
     Diagnosis, laboratory   3
       Nursing practice   239
     Genetics   9
     Governmental agencies
      119, 423
     Health sciences   119
       Management   120
     Instruments   119
     Journals
       Healthline   243
       Medicine   3, 340
       Medline   243
       Popline   243
       Sciences   340
       Social sciences   340
     Medical orders   18, 313
     Medicine   3, 9, 119, 120,
      134, 260, 279, 313
     Occupational therapy   3
     Ophthalmology   323
     Organizations, medical   3,
      119
     Orthopedics   254
     Pharmacology   9
     Physical therapy   3
     Physiology   9, 378
     Sciences   9

ABDOMEN

     See also specific organs
    RT   Gastrointestinal system
    RT   Genitourinary system
     Treatment, immunotherapy
      4
     Treatment, surgical
       Chemotherapy   4
       History   4
       Incisions   4
       Indications   4
       Nutrition   4
       Shock   4
       Techniques   4

ABNORMALITIES

     See Diseases

ABORTION

    RT   Gynecology
    RT   Obstetrics
    RT   Pregnancy
     Indications   191
     Legal aspects   191
     Nursing practice   214, 258
     Pathology
       Gynecology   310
       Obstetrics   310
     Sexuality
       Nursing practice   214
       Psychological aspects
        89
     Techniques   89, 191

ABSORPTION AND FATE (DRUGS)

     See Pharmacokinetics

UF-Used For, BT-Broader Term, NT-Narrower Term, RT-Related Term

ABSTRACT SERVICES

    RT   Abstracts, literature
    RT   Indexing services
    Journals   420
    Journals, nursing   34

ABSTRACTS, LITERATURE

    RT   Abstract services
    RT   Indexes, literature
    Chromosomal anomalies   69
    Teratogenic agents
        Chemicals   64
        Drugs   64
        Physical factors   64
        Viruses   64

ACADEMIC CALENDARS

    UF   Timetables, academic
    BT   Calendars
    Allied health sciences
        schools   13
    Dental schools   10
    Medical schools   1, 275

ACCIDENTS

    NT   Burns
    NT   Choking
    RT   Critical care
    RT   Emergency care
    RT   Injuries
    Aged   72
    Medicolegal investigations
        292
    Mortality
        Statistical data   437
    Pediatrics
        Treatment   108, 109
    Public health
        Epidemiology   259
        Prevention   259
    Tabular data
        Signs and symptoms   286
        Treatment   286

ACCREDITATION

    Standards
        Allied health sciences
            schools   13
        Hospitals   6
    Statistical data
        Nursing schools   308

Status
    Hospitals   184

ACID-BASE BALANCE

    RT   Acid-base disturbances
    RT   Body fluids
    RT   Buffers
    Anesthesia   233
    Respiratory system   117

ACID-BASE DISTURBANCES

    RT   Acid-base balance
    RT   Diseases
    RT   Electrolyte distur-
         bances
    Kidney
        Diagnosis   236
        Pathophysiology   236
        Signs and symptoms   236
        Treatment   236
    Nursing practice
        Case histories   314
        Diagnosis, laboratory
            314
        Signs and symptoms   314

ACRONYMS

    RT   Abbreviations
    RT   Initialisms
    Allied health sciences
        260
    Biochemistry   9
    Biology   209
    Dentistry   216
    Drugs, new   422
    Genetics   9
    Governmental agencies
        423
    Management
        Health sciences   120
    Medicine   9, 134, 260
    Organizations   147
    Pharmacology   9
    Physiology   9
    Sciences   9

ACTIONS AND USES

    UF   Indications
    RT   Pharmacokinetics
    Drugs   15, 18, 20, 50, 55,
        136, 138, 158, 175, 257,
        285, 371, 428, 429

Nursing practice 137,
160, 312, 313
Patient education 280,
427
Veterinary medicine 51,
434
Drugs, European 257
Durgs, immunosuppressive
73
Drugs, new 138
Drugs, nonprescription
349
Drugs (treatment modality)
Cardiovascular diseases
Nursing practice 62
Communicable diseases
354, 355
Emergency care
Nursing practice 144
Mental illness 189
Oral diseases 5
Veterinary diseases 435
Plants, medicinal 247
Vitamins 175

ACTUARIAL TABLES

See Life tables

ADDRESSES

RT Directories
RT Telephone numbers
Administrators
Health care services
184, 440
Hospitals 123
Allied health sciences
schools 13, 261, 341
American Medical Associa-
tion
Committee members 14
Staff members 14
Trustees 14
Archives 129
Audiovisual producers 90
Authors
Periodical literature
102, 103, 383
Proceedings, published
221
Biological scientists 23
Boards of nursing 296
Boards of pharmacy, state
136
Burn centers 296

Cancer research institutes
230
Cancer treatment centers
230
Cancer treatment programs
86
Certifying boards
Dental licensure 17
Consultants
Health care 261
Dental schools 10, 36,
216, 341
Executive search firms
362
Federal job information
centers 129
Foundations 164
Directories 163
Funeral service schools
389
Governmental agencies 90,
151, 261, 299, 423
Grants 261
Hospitals 184, 261, 317,
424
Hospitals, Canada 58
Hospitals, United Kingdom
268
Information centers 129
Information services 150
Information systems 150
Insurance companies 90
Investigators
Cancer protocols, exper-
imental 87
Health research awards
374
Laboratories 424
Libraries for the blind
129, 261
Libraries, medical 125,
129, 261
Libraries, research 129
Libraries, special 129
Libraries, world 445
Manufacturers, chemicals
68, 85
Manufacturers, drugs 18,
19, 136, 348, 349, 429
Manufacturers, drugs,
European 257
Manufacturers, drugs,
veterinary medicine 434
Manufacturers, equipment,
medical 263
Manufacturers, health

care products, Canada 58
Manufacturers, laboratory
  equipment 183
Manufacturers, laboratory
  instruments 183
Manufacturers, medical
  devices 267
Manufacturers, medical
  products 263
Medical examination
  boards, state 424
Medical licensing boards,
  state 424
Medical schools 1, 2, 36,
  261, 275, 341, 424
Medical schools, foreign
  36, 261, 442
Medical schools, United
  Kingdom 268
Medical specialists 126
Members
  American College of Phy-
    sicians 45
  American College of Sur-
    geons 16
  American Dental Associa-
    tion 17
  American Hospital Asso-
    ciation 184
  American Psychiatry
    Association 44
  American Public Health
    Association 46
  Congressional subcommit-
    tees 299
Multihospital systems 184
Museums, world 445
Nursing homes 424
Nursing schools 341
Officials
  American Dental Associa-
    tion 17
  American Medical Associ-
    ation 14
Organizations
  Directories 446
Organizations, dental 17,
  151
Organizations, dental,
  state
  Officials 17
Organizations, medical
  58, 147, 151, 198, 261,
  385
Organizations, nursing
  151, 157, 246, 296

Organizations, patient
  education 90
Organizations, pharmacol-
  ogic 136, 151
Organizations, scientific
  147, 385
Patent depository librar-
  ies 129
Pediatrics
  Health care services
    297
  Mental health services
    297
  Treatment facilities
    297
Pharmacists 343
Pharmacy schools 341
Physical scientists 23
Physicians 22, 130, 424
Physicians, United Kingdom
  268, 274
Physicians, women 130
Poison control centers
  225, 246, 261, 296, 348,
  349
Public health schools 46,
  341
Public health scientists
  23
Publishers
  Books, in print 53, 265
  Journals 34, 102, 103,
    261, 265, 268, 420
Research centers 375
Research institutes, for-
  eign 445
Research programs
  Allied health sciences
    376
  Dentistry 376
  Medicine 376
  Pharmacology 376
  Veterinary medicine 376
Residency programs, ac-
  credited 128
Runaway youth centers 297
Senators and representa-
  tives 299
Universities, world 445
Veterinary medicine
  schools 341
Voluntary health organiza-
  tions 90

ADMINISTRATION (DRUGS)

See Dosage and administration

ADMINISTRATION, HOSPITAL

See Hospital administra-
tion

ADMINISTRATORS

NT Hospital administrators
RT Chairpersons
RT Contact persons
RT Deans
RT Department heads
RT Directors
RT Executives
RT Officials
Health care services   440
Hospitals 184, 424
Medical schools, United
 Kingdom 268
Nursing homes   424

ADMISSION REQUIREMENTS

Allied health sciences
 schools 13
Dental schools   10, 36
Medical schools 36, 275
Medical schools, foreign
 36

ADMISSION STATISTICS

Dental schools 36
Hospitals 58, 184, 212,
 443
Medical schools 36
Medical schools, foreign
 442
Nursing schools 308

ADOLESCENCE

UF Teenagers
RT Pediatrics
Alcohol abuse
 Treatment 109
Drug abuse
 Treatment 109
Family medicine 406
Gynecology 106
 Anatomy 186
 Diseases
   Signs and symptoms

186
 Treatment 186
 Embryology 186
 History and physical ex-
  amination 186
 Physiology 186
 Pregnancy 266
 Sexuality 109, 186
Hypertension 78
Nutrition 293
Patient education   21

ADOPTION

Directories 381

ADRENALS

BT Endocrine system
RT Hormones
Anatomy 57
Diseases
 Diagnosis 57
 Signs and symptoms   57
 Treatment   57
Physiology 57

ADVERSE EFFECTS

NT Carcinogenicity
NT Drug interactions
NT Interferences
RT Complications
RT Overdosage
RT Teratogenic agents
RT Toxicology
RT Warnings
Antibiotic drugs 105
Antimicrobial drugs   105
Biological hazards   319
Chemical constituents
 Body fluids 105
Chemical hazards   319
Diets, modified   187
Drugs 15, 20, 136, 138,
 156, 158, 175, 188, 289,
 350, 371, 428
 Bibliographies 289
 Nursing practice 137,
  160, 312, 313
 Patient education   21,
  280, 427
 Veterinary medicine   434
Drugs, European   257
Drugs, new   344
Drugs, prescription 348

UF-Used For, BT-Broader Term, NT-Narrower Term, RT-Related Term

Drugs (treatment modality)
 Diseases   30
  Allergy   12
  Communicable diseases
   355
  Nursing practice   62,
   160, 295
  Oral diseases   5
  Pediatrics
   Emergency care   412
  Rheumatology   31, 414
  Veterinary medicine
   435
 Immunizations   253
  Communicable diseases
   354
 Pesticides   319
 Physical hazards   319
 Prevention
  Anesthesia, regional
   238
 Treatment
  Anesthesia, regional
   238
  Cancer   61

ADVERTISEMENTS

 UF Announcements
 Residency training pro-
  grams   178

AGED

 UF Elderly
 UF Geriatrics
 UF Old age
 Accidents   72
 Anesthesia   233
  Pathophysiology   28
 Biology   72
 Death and dying   72
 Dentistry   72
 Diseases
  Diagnosis   72
  Treatment   72
 Drugs   72, 188
 Encyclopedias, loose-
  leaf   81
 Health care services   203,
  381
 Hormones   405
 Long-term care   72
 Nutrition   293
 Patient education   21
 Physiology   72, 272

Sexuality   72

AGENCIES, GOVERNMENTAL

 See Governmental agencies

AGENCIES, HOME HEALTH

 See Home health agencies

AIR POLLUTION

 RT   Ecology
 RT   Environmental health
 RT   Noise pollution
 RT   Radiation pollution
 Industrial control   114
 Industrial hazards   114
 Toxicology
  Pharmacology   175
  Signs and symptoms   175
  Treatment   175

ALCOHOL ABUSE

 BT   Drug abuse
 Adolescence
  Treatment   109
 Treatment programs
  Directories   203

ALCOHOL USE

 Behavioral factors   259

ALCOHOLIC BEVERAGES

 UF   Beverages, alcoholic
 BT   Beverages
 RT   Foods
 Composition   54, 245

ALGAE

 BT   Plants
 RT   Strains, algae
 Tabular data   98

ALIMENTARY TRACT

 NT   Anus
 NT   Colon
 NT   Duodenum
 NT   Esophagus
 NT   Gastrointestinal system
 NT   Mouth

NT   Rectum
NT   Stomach
Diseases
   Treatment, surgical   393

ALLERGIC RESPONSE

   Induction   73
   Physiology   73

ALLERGY

   RT   Immunology
   Diseases
      Diagnosis   12, 250
      Drugs (treatment modali-
      ty)
         Adverse effects   12
         Dosage and administra-
            tion   12
         Pharmacokinetics   12
         Pharmacology   12
         Toxicology   12
      Signs and symptoms   12
   Encyclopedias, loose-leaf
      81
   Hormones   405
   Immunology   12
   Pathology   388
   Physiology   12, 388

ALLIED HEALTH SCIENCES

   RT   Allied health sciences
      schools
   Abbreviations   260
   Acronyms   260
   Dictionaries   52, 145
   Directories
      Bibliographies   124
   Encyclopedias   145
   Indexes, literature   218,
      315
   Reference books
      Bibliographies, anno-
         tated   201
   Research programs
      Directories   376
   Thesauri   262

ALLIED HEALTH SCIENCES
SCHOOLS

   UF   Education, allied
        health sciences
   BT   University programs

RT   Allied health sciences
Directories
   Academic calendars   13
   Accreditation   13
   Addresses   13, 261, 341
   Admission requirements
      13
   Affiliates   13
   Certificates awarded   13
   Chairpersons   341
   Deans   261
   Degrees awarded   13
   Faculty, number of   341
   Financial aid   13
   Programs offered   341
   Students, number of   341
   Telephone numbers   13,
      261, 341
   Tuition   13, 341
   University community
      341
Information sources   13
Statistical data   13

ALMANACS

   RT   Handbooks
   RT   Statistical data
   RT   Tabular data
   Nursing practice   438
   Pediatrics   439

AMA EVALUATIONS

   Drugs   15

AMBULATORY MEDICINE

   RT   Outpatient surgery
   RT   Outpatient visits
   Diseases
      Diagnosis   358
      Epidemiology   358
      Etiology   358
      Pathogenesis   358
      Physical examination   358
      Prognosis   358
      Signs and symptoms   358
      Treatment   358
   Pediatrics   108

AMERICAN BOARD OF SURGERY

   BT   American specialty
        boards
   BT   Organizations, medical

Examinations   415

AMERICAN COLLEGE OF PHYSI-
CIANS

BT   Organizations, medical
RT   Physicians
 Members
  Addresses   45
  Awards   45
  Birth dates   45
  Birth places   45
  Educational backgrounds
   45
  Marriage dates   45
  Professional activities
   5
  Professional certifica-
   tions   45
  Specialties   45
  Spouses   45
  Telephone numbers   45
 Officials   45
 Organizational handbooks
  45
 Pledges (text)   45

AMERICAN COLLEGE OF SURGEONS

BT   Organizations, medical
RT   Physicians
 Members
  Addresses   16
  Birth dates   16
  Dates of membership   16
  Educational backgrounds
   16
  Professional certifica-
   tions   16
  Professional memberships
   16
  Specialties   16
 Officials   16
 Organizational handbooks
  16

AMERICAN DENTAL ASSOCIATION

UF   Dentists
BT   Organizations, dental
 Members
  Addresses   17
  Birth dates   17
  Educational backgrounds
   17
  Membership status   17

Officials
  Addresses   17
 Functions   216
 Organization   216
 Standards
  Dental care
   Hospitals   210

AMERICAN HOSPITAL ASSOCIATION

BT   Organizations, medical
 Awards   184
 Members
  Addresses   184
 Officials   184

AMERICAN MEDICAL ASSOCIATION

BT   Organizations, medical
RT   Physicians
 Committee members
  Addresses   14
  Telephone numbers   14
 Officials
  Addresses   14
  Telephone numbers   14
 Staff members
  Addresses   14
  Telephone numbers   14
 Trustees
  Addresses   14
  Telephone numbers   14

AMERICAN PSYCHIATRY ASSOCIA-
TION

UF   Psychiatrists
BT   Organizations, medical
RT   Physicians
 Members
  Addresses   44
  Birth dates   44
  Certification   44
  Educational backgrounds
   44
  Employment status   44
  Hospital affiliations
   44
  Professional activities
   44
  Professional memberships
   44
  Publications   44
  Telephone numbers   44
 Officials   44
 Pledges (text)   44

AMERICAN PUBLIC HEALTH ASSO-
CIATION

BT   Organizations, medical
Members
   Addresses   46
   Awards   46
   Birth dates   46
   Birth places   46
   Educational backgrounds
   46
   Professional certifica-
   tions   46
   Professional experience
   46
   Telephone numbers   46
Organizational handbooks
46

AMERICAN SPECIALTY BOARDS

UF   Medical specialists
BT   Organizations, medical
NT   American Board of Sur-
   gery
RT   Physicians
RT   Specialists
Eligibility requirements
126
Functions   126
History   126
Members   126
Officials   126
Purposes   126

AMINO ACIDS

RT   Peptides
RT   Polypeptides
RT   Proteins
Biochemistry
   Biosynthesis   43
   Tabular data   94
Microbial composition
   Tabular data   98
Nutritional content
   Foods   54, 245

AMPUTATIONS

See Orthopedics

ANALGESIA

See Anesthesia

ANATOMICAL TABLES

RT   Anatomy
Arteries   52, 145, 283
Bones   52, 145, 283
Muscles   52, 145, 283
Nerves   52, 145, 283
Synovial joints   52
Veins   52, 145, 283

ANATOMY

NT   Histology
RT   Anatomical tables
RT   Morphology
RT   Physiology
RT   Positions, anatomical
Adrenals   57
Alimentary tract
   Treatment, surgical   393
Anesthesia, regional   238
Animals   146
Anus
   Treatment, surgical   394
Athletic injuries   419
Atlases   25, 70, 180, 296
Bile ducts   132
Biliary tract   133
Blood vessels   205
Body parts   181, 402
Body systems   181, 402
Cancer   7
Cardiovascular system
   Nursing practice   62
   Treatment, surgical   417
Classification systems
347
Colon
   Treatment, surgical   394
Critical care
   Nursing practice   100
Dermatology   116
Diagnosis, radiologic   174
Endocrine system   405
Gallbladder   132
Gastrointestinal system
168, 169
Genitourinary system   57,
172
Genitourinary system, fe-
male   185
   Embryology   191
Gynecology   106, 311, 318
   Adolescence   186
   Nursing practice   258
   Pediatrics   186

UF-Used For, BT-Broader Term, NT-Narrower Term, RT-Related Term

Head
  Treatment, surgical   32
Heart   205
History and physical exam-
  ination   174
Kidneys   236
Liver   132, 133
Neck
  Treatment, surgical   32
Nervous system   92
  Nursing practice   63
Nomenclature   180, 309
Obstetrics   441
  Treatment, surgical   321
Ophthalmology   171, 323
  Nursing practice   316
Orthopedics   254
  Diseases   327
  Fractures   327
Otolaryngology   328, 411
  Nursing practice   316
Patient education   21
Plastic surgery   369
Rectum
  Treatment, surgical   394
Respiratory system   117,
  365
Rheumatology   31
Sexuality   89
Thorax
  Treatment, surgical   417
Treatment, surgical
  Atlases   24
Veterinary medicine   309

ANEMIA

  RT Hematology
  Differential diagnosis
  244

ANESTHESIA

  UF Analgesia
  NT Anesthesia, regional
  RT Anesthesia practice,
      consultant
  RT Treatment, surgical
  Acid-base balance   233
  Aged   233
    Pathophysiology   28
  Cardiopulmonary resuscita-
    tion   233
  Cardiopulmonary surgery
    233
  Complications   233

Controlled hypotension
  233
Diseases
  Pathophysiology   28
Emergency care
  Pathophysiology   28
Equipment   233
Heart   205, 206
Infants   233
  Pathophysiology   28
Intravenous fluids   233
Obesity
  Pathophysiology   28
Obstetrics   321
Outpatient surgery   233
Pain control   233
Pediatrics   233
  Agent selection   29
  Blood replacement   29
  Complications   29
  Dentistry   29
  Fluid therapy   29
  Intensive care   29
  Legal aspects   29
  Monitoring   29
  Mortality   29
  Techniques   29
  Treatment, surgical
    29
Postoperative care   233
Pregnancy
  Pathophysiology   28
Preoperative preparation
  233
Techniques   27, 233
Tracheal intubation   233
Treatment, surgical
  Agent selection   27
  Diseases   360
    Cardiovascular system
    417
    Thorax   417
  Equipment   27
  Face   409
  Handbooks   110
  Maxilla   409
  Mouth   409
  Nervous system   233
  Nursing care   11
  Obstetrics   321
  Ophthalmology   322
  Oral diseases   409
  Patient care   27
  Pharmacology   27
  Techniques   27, 233

ANESTHESIA PRACTICE, CONSULT-
ANT

   RT   Anesthesia
   Cardiopulmonary resuscita-
    tion 27
   Intensive care   27
   Pain control   27
   Pulmonary function testing
    27
   Respiratory care   27

ANESTHESIA, REGIONAL

   BT   Anesthesia
   Adverse effects
    Prevention   238
    Treatment   238
   Anatomy   238
   Atlases   238
   Techniques   238

ANIMAL CELL LINES

   UF   Cell lines, animal
   Catalogs
    Cultures   66

ANIMAL HOSTS

   RT   Parasitology
   Diseases
    Handbooks   97

ANIMALS

   NT   Animals, marine
   NT   Cats
   NT   Cattle
   NT   Dogs
   NT   Horses
   NT   Pigs
   NT   Sheep
   NT   Small animals
   RT   Laboratory animal
    sciences
   RT   Veterinary medicine
   Classification systems
    209
   Common names   48
   Diseases
    Diagnosis   131
    Treatment   131
   Encyclopedias
    Anatomy   146

Diseases   146
Genetics   146
Parasitology   146
Pregnancy
   Diagnosis   146
Viruses
   Classification systems
   146
   Nomenclature   146
Poisoning (of humans)
   Diagnosis   193, 351
   Prevention   193
   Prognosis   193
   Signs and symptoms   193,
    351
   Treatment   193, 351
Scientific names   48

ANIMALS, MARINE

   BT   Animals
   NT   Fish
   Illustrations   352
   Poisoning (of humans)
    Biology   352
    Chemistry   352
    Geographical distribu-
     tion   352
    Illustrations   352
    Nomenclatures   352
    Pathology   352
    Pharmacology   352
    Prevention   352
    Signs and symptoms   352
    Toxicology   352
    Treatment   352

ANNOUNCEMENTS

   See Advertisements

ANNUAL REPORTS

   Secretary of Health & Hu-
    man Services   204
    Health status   204
    Health trends   204

ANOMALIES, CHROMOSOMAL

   See Chromosomal anomalies

ANTEPARTAL CARE

   RT   Childbirth
   RT   Obstetrics

UF–Used For, BT–Broader Term, NT–Narrower Term, RT–Related Term

Nursing practice 258

ANTIBIOTIC DRUGS

  BT Drugs
  Actions and uses 354
  Adverse effects 105
  Dosage and administration
    105, 354
  Indications 105
  Pharmacology 105
  Routes of administration
    105

ANTIMICROBIAL DRUGS

  BT Drugs
  Adverse effects 105
  Dosage and administration
    105
  Indications 105
  Pharmacology 105
  Routes of administration
    105

ANUS

  BT Alimentary tract
  BT Gastrointestinal system
  Diseases
    Signs and symptoms 394
    Treatment, surgical
      393, 394

APHASIAS

  Neurology
    Encyclopedias, loose-
      leaf 82

ARCHITECTS

  Health care
    Directories 381

ARCHIVES

  RT Libraries, special
  Directories
    Addresses 129
    Directors 129
    Founding dates 129
    Holdings
      Statistical data 129
    Networks and consortia
      129

Publications 129
Services 129
Special collections 129
Staff names 129
Staff, number of 129
Subjects 129
Telephone numbers 129

ARTERIES

  BT Cardiovascular system
  RT Blood
  RT Hematology
  RT Vascular diseases
  RT Veins
  Anatomical tables 52,
    145, 283

ARTHRITIS

  See Rheumatology

ARTHRODESIS

  Orthopedics 56

ARTHROPLASTY

  Orthopedics 56

ARTHROPODS

  UF Spiders
  RT Bites and stings
  RT Parasitology
  Biology 83
  Classification systems 83
  Diagnosis, immunologic 83
  Diseases
    Diagnosis 83
    Epidemiology 83
    Pathogenesis 83
    Pathology 83
    Prevention 83
    Prognosis 83
    Signs and symptoms 83
    Treatment 83
  Entomologic methods 83
  History 83
  Illustrations 83
  Life cycles 83
  Morphology 83
  Specimen examination tech-
    niques 83

ASPHYXIAL DEATHS

BT   Death and dying
  Medicolegal investigations
  292

ASSAYS

  BT   Tests
  RT   Laboratory techniques
  Bacteriology
    Microbiology 251
  Chemicals, European   155
  Drugs   426
  Fungi
    Microbiology 251
  Parasitology
    Microbiology 251
  Pharmaceutical ingredients
  426
  Rickettsiae
    Microbiology 251
  Spirochetes
    Microbiology 251
  Viruses
    Microbiology 251

ASSESSMENT

  See Diagnosis

ASSOCIATION OF AMERICAN MEDI-
CAL COLLEGES

  BT   Organizations, medical
  RT   Medical schools
  Directories
    Activities   2
    Awards   2
    Members 2
    Officials 2

ASSOCIATION OF CANCER CENTERS

  BT   Organizations, medical
  Delegate rosters   86

ASSOCIATIONS

  See Organizations

ATHLETIC INJURIES

  UF   Sports injuries
  BT   Injuries
  Anatomy 419
  Diagnosis 419
  Prevention 419

Rehabilitation   419
Treatment   419

ATLASES

RT   Identification
RT   Illustrations
Abdomen
  Treatment, surgical   4
Alimentary tract
  Treatment, surgical   393
Anatomy   25, 70, 180, 296
  Treatment, surgical   24,
  379
Anesthesia, regional   238
Anus
  Treatment, surgical   394
Birth defects   49, 69
Blood
  Histology 33
Cardiovascular system
  Treatment, surgical   417
Chromosomal anomalies   69
Colon
  Treatment, surgical   394
Dermatology
  Handbooks 256
Diagnosis
  Procedures 70
Diseases   70
  Dermatology   116
  Gross characteristics
  8
Drugs 136
Embryology 269
Epithelium
  Histology 33
Head
  Radiographic anatomy 32
  Treatment, surgical 32
Hematology
  Diagnosis, laboratory
  240
Histology 33
  Diseases 8
History and physical exam-
  ination 181
Identification
  Pathogenic microorganisms
  35
Instruments, surgical
  Nursing practice 228
Integument
  Histology 33
Neck
  Radiographic anatomy 32

UF-Used For, BT-Broader Term, NT-Narrower Term, RT-Related Term

Treatment, surgical   32
Obstetrics
  Treatment, surgical   321
Orthopedics
  Birth fractures
    Diagnosis   115
    Mechanism of injury
      115
    Treatment   115
  Dislocations
    Diagnosis   115
    Mechanism of injury   115
    Treatment   115
  Fracture-dislocations
    Diagnosis   115
    Mechanism of injury   115
    Treatment   115
  Fractures
    Diagnosis   115
    Mechanism of injury   115
    Treatment   115
  Subluxations
    Diagnosis   115
    Mechanism of injury   115
    Treatment   115
  Physiology   70
  Plants, medicinal   247
  Rectum
    Treatment, surgical   394
  Thorax
    Treatment, surgical   417
  Treatment, surgical
    Anatomy   24, 379

ATOMIC WEIGHTS

  BT   Weights and measures
  Drugs, European   257

AUDIOVISUAL MATERIALS

  UF   Films
  UF   Slides
  UF   Tapes
  UF   Videorecordings
  Catalogs
    National Library of Med-
      icine   300
  Producers
    Directories   90
  Toxicology   225

AUTHORS

  NT   Writers, medical
  Books   53, 265, 302

Periodical literature
  Addresses   102, 103, 383
Proceedings, published
  221

AUTHORS' GUIDES

  RT   Proofreading marks
  RT   Publishing, medical
  RT   Style manuals
  RT   Writing, medical
  Journals, nursing   34

AUTOPSIES

  UF   Necropsies
  RT   Causes of death
  RT   Death and dying
  Techniques   292
  Veterinary medicine   432

AWARDS

  American College of Physi-
    cians   45
  American Hospital Associa-
    tion   184
  American Public Health
    Association   46
  Association of American
    Medical Colleges   2
  Health care   198, 381
  Hospital administrators
    123
  Medicine   261
  Nursing   303

BACTERIOLOGY

  BT   Microbiology
  RT   Rickettsiae
  RT   Spirochetes
  RT   Strains
  RT   Strains, bacteria
  Assays   251
  Biochemistry   39
  Catalogs
    Reference strains   39
    Strains   65
    Type strains   39
  Characterization   251
  Classification systems
    39, 251
  Culture and isolation   251
  Diagnosis, laboratory
    179, 251

Reagents 179
Ecology 39
Examination 251
Genetic data 39
Graduate schools
  Ratings 176
Identification 251
Illustrations
  Indexes 39
Media formulas 179
Nomenclature 39, 251
Nutrition 39
Physiology 39
Serodiagnosis 251
Stain formulas 179
Staining techniques 179
Tabular data 98, 99
Taxonomy 251
Tests 179, 251
Undergraduate schools
  Ratings 177

BARNES HOSPITAL

Normal laboratory values
253

BASSINETS, NUMBER OF

BT Beds, number of
Hospitals 184

BATTERED WOMEN SERVICES

UF Wife abuse
Directories 203

BEDS, NUMBER OF

NT Bassinets, number of
NT Burn beds
Hospitals 58, 128, 184,
  212, 268, 317, 424, 443
Nursing homes 424

BEHAVIORAL SCIENCES

NT Psychiatry
RT Mental illness
Indexes, literature 383
  Review articles 222
U.S. government documents
  Indexes 282

BEREAVEMENT COUNSELING

Death and dying 389

BEVERAGES

NT Alcoholic beverages
RT Foods
Caffeine content 54, 187
Composition 245

BEVERAGES, ALCOHOLIC

See Alcoholic beverages

BIBLIOGRAPHIES

NT Bibliographies, anno-
    tated
RT Indexes, literature
RT Information sources
Adverse effects
  Drugs 289
Bioethics 41
Directories
  Allied health sciences
  124
  Dentistry 124
  Health care 124
  Medicine 124
  Nursing 124
  Pharmacology 124
  Sciences 124
  Veterinary medicine 124
Diseases
  History 42
  Mendelian inheritance
  284
Ethics, medical 41
Medicine
  Biography 42
  History 42
Original articles
  Diagnostic techniques
  152
  Diseases 152, 217, 368
  Strains 152
  Syndromes 121, 217, 368
  Treatment, surgical 42,
  152
Proceedings, published
  127, 221, 361
Reference books 162

BIBLIOGRAPHIES, ANNOTATED

BT Bibliographies
RT Indexes, literature

History
  Diseases 264
  Ethics, medical 264
  Public health 264
  Toxicology 264
  Treatment, surgical 264
Patient education 90
Reference books 182, 201,
  273
Toxicology
  Chemicals 370

BILE DUCTS

  NT Biliary ducts, extra-
        hepatic
  RT Gallbladder
  RT Liver
  Anatomy 132, 133
  Diseases
    Diagnosis 132, 133
    Pathology 133
    Signs and symptoms 132,
      133
    Treatment 132, 133
  Embryology 132

BILIARY DUCTS, EXTRAHEPATIC

  BT Bile ducts
  RT Gallbladder
  Diseases
    Treatment, surgical 393

BILL OF RIGHTS, DYING PERSONS

  RT Patient rights
  Nursing practice 438

BILL OF RIGHTS, PATIENTS

  RT Patient rights
  Nursing practice 438

BILL OF RIGHTS, PREGNANT
PATIENTS

  RT Patient rights
  Nursing practice 438

BIOCHEMISTRY

  BT Chemistry
  Abbreviations 9, 43
  Acronyms 9
  Amino acids

    Tabular data 94
Bacteriology 39
Biosynthesis
  Amino acids 43
  Carbohydrates 43
  Lipids 43
  Nucleotides 43
Body fluid disturbances
  74
Buffers
    Tabular data 94
Carbohydrates
    Tabular data 94
Catabolism 43
Cells 43
Chromatography
    Tabular data 94
CRC handbooks
    Indexes 93
Diseases 415
    Pathophysiology 403
Electrolyte disturbances
  74
Endocrine system 153, 403
Enzymes 43, 403
Genetics 43
Graduate schools
    Ratings 176
Handbooks 94
Hematology 77, 207
History, chronological 43
Hormone action 43
Initialisms 9
Ion exchange
    Tabular data 94
Liver 132
Metabolism 403
Motile system 43
Muscles 43
Nucleic acids
    Tabular data 94
Nucleotides
    Tabular data 94
Nutrition 403
Oligonucleotides
    Tabular data 94
Ophthalmology 323
Origin of life 43
Otolaryngology 328
Peptides
    Tabular data 94
Polypeptides
    Tabular data 94
Pregnancy
    Complications 266
Proteins   43

Tabular data   94
Purines
  Tabular data   94
Pyrimidines
  Tabular data   94
Respiratory system   413
Steroids
  Tabular data   94
Undergraduate schools
  Ratings   177
Vitamins
  Tabular data   94

BIOETHICS

See Ethics, medical

BIOGRAPHIES

RT   Directories
Administrators
  Health care services
  440
Bibliographies   42
Physicians   47, 234

BIOLOGICAL REGULATORS

Tabular data   48

BIOLOGICAL SCIENCES SCHOOLS

UF   Education, biological
     sciences
BT   University programs
RT   Biology
Addresses   341
Chairpersons   341
Expenses   341
Faculty, number of   341
Programs offered   341
Students, number of   341
Telephone numbers   341
University community   341

BIOLOGICAL SCIENTISTS

BT   Scientists
RT   Biology
Addresses   23
Birth dates   23
Educational backgrounds
23
Marriage dates   23
Memberships   23
Professional experience

23
Specialties   23

BIOLOGICALS

Prices (retail & whole-
sale)
  Drug store merchandise
  136

BIOLOGY

NT   Cell biology
NT   Cytology
NT   Molecular biology
RT   Biological sciences
     schools
RT   Biological scientists
Abbreviations   209
Acronyms   209
Aged   72
Animal kingdom
  Classification systems
  209
Arthropods
  Parasitology   83
Dermatology   116
Dictionaries   209
Engineering
  CRC handbooks   93
Helminths
  Parasitology   83
Human behavior   89
Plant kingdom
  Classification systems
  209
Poisoning
  Animals, marine   352
Protozoa
  Parasitology   83
Ratings
  Graduate schools   176
  Undergraduate schools
  177
Tabular data
  Biological regulators
  48
  Biomechanics   96
  Body fluids   48
  Chemical constants   48
  Circulation   48
  Culture media   48
  Cytology   48
  Digestion   48
  Electronics   96
  Engineering   96

UF-Used For, BT-Broader Term, NT-Narrower Term, RT-Related Term

Environment 48
Excretion 48
Genetics 48
Growth and development
 48
Laboratory materials 48
Mathematical constants
 48
Metabolism 48
Neurobiology 48
Nutrition 48
Parasitology 48
Physiological constants
 48
Reproduction 48
Respiration 48
Taxonomy 48
Toxins, animal 48
Toxins, plant 48

BIOMECHANICS

Biology
  Tabular data 96
Medicine
  Tabular data 96

BIOSYNTHESIS

Biochemistry
  Amino acids 43
  Carbohydrates 43
  Lipids 43
  Nucleotides 43

BIRTH

See Childbirth

BIRTH CONTROL

See Contraception

BIRTH DATES

BT Dates
Administrators
  Health care services
  440
Biological scientists 23
Hospital administrators
 123
Medical specialists 126
Members
  American College of
  Physicians 45

American College of
  Surgeons 16
American Dental Associa-
  tion 17
American Psychiatry As-
  sociation 44
American Public Health
  Association 46
Congressional subcommit-
  tees 299
Pharmacists 343
Physical scientists 23
Physicians 424
Public health scientists
 23

BIRTH DEFECTS

UF Congenital anomalies
RT Chromosomal anomalies
RT Teratology
Atlases 49
Carrier detection 49
Complications 49
Diagnosis 49
Etiology 49
Mendelian inheritance,
 mode of 49
Metabolic diseases 49
Obstetrics 321
Pathogenesis 49
Pediatrics
  Classification systems
  339
  Screening 339
Prognosis 49
Signs and symptoms 49
Treatment 49

BIRTH FRACTURES

BT Fractures
RT Childbirth
RT Orthopedics
Diagnosis
  Atlases 115
Mechanism of injury
  Atlases 115
Treatment
  Atlases 115

BIRTH PLACES

Hospital administrators
 123
Members

American College of Physicians 45
American Public Health Association 46
Congressional subcommittees 299
Specialists 126

BIRTHS, NUMBER OF

BT Vital statistics
RT Natality
Hospitals 58, 184

BITES AND STINGS

UF Insect bites and stings
NT Snakebites
RT Arthropods
RT Poisoning
Diagnosis 193, 351
Emergency care
  Nursing practice 144
Etiology 196
Immunizations 37
Prevention 193
Prognosis 193
Signs and symptoms 111, 193, 196, 286, 351
  Pediatrics 304
Treatment 111, 193, 196, 286, 351
  Pediatrics 109, 304

BLEEDING

NT Gastrointestinal bleeding
RT Hematology
Differential diagnosis 244

BLIND SERVICES

BT Handicapped services
Directories 203

BLOOD

RT Arteries
RT Cardiovascular system
RT Hematology
RT Serodiagnosis
RT Spleen
RT Vascular diseases

RT Veins
Atlases
  Histology 33
Body fluids
  Physiology 40
Chemical constituents 52
Normal laboratory values 77, 144
Pathophysiology 331

BLOOD BANKS

Directories 381
Tabular data 99

BLOOD GASES

Respiratory system 117

BLOOD PRESSURE

RT Hypertension
Pediatrics 195

BLOOD STORAGE

Pediatrics 208

BLOOD TRANSFUSIONS

Hematology 360
  Pediatrics 208
    Anesthesia 29

BOARDS OF NURSING

UF Nursing boards
Addresses 296
Telephone numbers 296

BOARDS OF PHARMACY, STATE

UF Pharmacy boards, state
Addresses 136
Contact persons 136
Telephone numbers 136

BODY COMPOSITION

Tabular data 170

BODY FLUID DISTURBANCES

RT Body fluids
RT Diseases
RT Electrolyte distur-

UF—Used For, BT—Broader Term, NT—Narrower Term, RT—Related Term

bances
Anesthesia
  Pediatrics   29
Biochemistry   74
Diagnosis   74, 236, 314
Nursing practice   314
Pathophysiology   74, 236
Physiology   74
Signs and symptoms   236,
  314
Treatment   74, 110, 236,
  360
    Pediatrics   397

BODY FLUIDS

  UF   Fluids, body
  RT   Acid-base balance
  RT   Body fluid disturbances
  RT   Electrolyte distur-
       bances
  Chemical constituents
    Adverse effects   105
  Pathology   330
  Physiology   272
    Blood   40
    Lymph   40
    Urine excretion   40
  Tabular data   48, 170
  Treatment, surgical   110

BODY PARTS, HUMAN

  See Human body parts

BODY SURFACE AREA

  Nomograms   110, 253, 418
    Pediatrics   192

BODY SYSTEMS, HUMAN

  See Human body systems

BONE MARROW

  Normal laboratory values
  77

BONES

  RT   Orthopedics
  Anatomical tables   52,
  145, 283

BOOKS

  BT   Publications
  NT   Books, in print
  NT   Books, 1876-1982
  NT   Reference books
  RT   Journals
  Catalogs
    National Library of Med-
      icine   302
  Classification systems
    Medicine   301

BOOKS, IN PRINT

  BT   Books
  Catalogs
    Ordering information
    53, 265

BOOKS, 1876-1982

  BT   Books
  Health care
    Catalogs   200
  Medicine
    Catalogs   200

BOTANICALS

  RT   Plants
  Prices (retail & whole-
    sale)
    Drug store merchandise
    136

BRAND NAMES

  UF   Names, brand
  UF   Proprietary names
  RT   Generic names
  RT   Trade names
  Chemical formulations   68
  Drugs   18, 20, 30, 138,
    158, 428, 429
    Nursing practice   313
  Drugs, European   257
  Drugs, new   138
  Drugs, nonprescription
    349
  Drugs, prescription   348
  Patient education
    Drugs   427

BREAST FEEDING

  UF   Lactation
  Drugs   20, 188, 232, 296,

428
Nursing practice   137
Patient education   427

BUFFERS

RT   Acid-base balance
Biochemistry
Tabular data   94

BURN BEDS, NUMBER OF

BT   Beds, number of
BT   Statistical data
Burn centers   296

BURN CENTERS

RT   Burns
Directories   296, 400

BURNS

BT   Accidents
RT   Burn centers
RT   Emergency care
RT   Fires
Nursing practice   100, 144
Pediatrics
Treatment   109
Signs and symptoms   111
Treatment   111, 136

BUYERS' GUIDES

RT   Catalogs
RT   Directories
Health care products,
Canada
Addresses   58
Contact persons   58
Telephone numbers   58

CAFFEINE CONTENT

RT   Nutrition
Beverages   54, 187

CALENDARS

NT   Academic calendars
Meetings, future, medical
Contact persons   386
Dates   386
Places   386
Sponsoring organizations

Addresses   386
Meetings, future, scien-
tific
Contact persons   386
Dates   386
Places   386
Sponsoring organizations
Addresses   386

CALL NUMBERS, NLM

Books   302
Journals   202, 219

CANADA

See terms below as thesaurus
entries for detailed infor-
mation
Archives   129
Burn centers   296
Dental schools   1, 10,
216, 275
Health care products
Buyers' guides   58
Health care services
Administrators   440
Hospitals, Canada   58
Information centers   129
Libraries, research   129
Libraries, special   129
Library networks   129
Manufacturers, medical de-
vices   267
Medical schools   1, 275,
424
Nursing practice
Law   241
Organizations   296
Organizations, medical   58
Poison control centers
246, 296

CANADIAN DENTAL ASSOCIATION

BT   Organizations, dental
Functions   216
Organizational structure
216

CANCER

UF   Neoplasms
UF   Oncology
BT   Diseases
Anatomy   7

UF-Used For, BT-Broader Term, NT-Narrower Term, RT-Related Term

Cell biology   61
Classification systems
  60
  Morphology   229
Complications, hematologic
  60
Complications, infections
  60
Diagnosis   7, 60, 61
Emergency care   61
Encyclopedias, loose-leaf
  81, 384
Epidemiology   7, 60, 61
Etiology   60, 61
Gynecology
  Radiation therapy   318
Pathogenesis   60
Pathology   7, 60, 61
Prevention   61
Prognosis   7, 60
Psychologic aspects   60
Psychosocial aspects   61
Public health
  Epidemiology   259
  Prevention   259
Rehabilitation   61
Signs and symptoms   7, 60
Staging   61
Statistical data   296
  Etiology   59
  Incidence   59
  Mortality   59
  Research   59
  Risk factors   59
  Survival   59
  Trends   59
Treatment   7
  Adverse effects   61
Treatment, chemicals   60,
  61
  Cross resistance   79
  Dosage and administra-
    tion   79
  Investigational agents
    79
  Toxicology   79
Treatment, endocrine   60
Treatment, experimental
  61
Treatment, immunotherapy
  60, 79
Treatment, radiation   60,
  61
Treatment, surgical   60,
  61

CANCER PROTOCOLS, EXPERIMEN-
  TAL

  UF   Protocols, cancer
  RT   Cancer treatment pro-
         grams
  RT   Investigational drugs
  RT   Treatment, chemicals
  RT   Treatment, experimental
  Dosage and administration
    87
  Entry criteria   87
  Investigators
    Addresses   87
    Telephone numbers   87
  Objectives   87
  Patient evaluation parame-
    ters   87
  Patients allowed in pro-
    gram, number   87
  Protocol outlines   87

CANCER RESEARCH INSTITUTES

  BT   Research centers
  RT   Research institutes,
         foreign
  RT   Research programs
  RT   Treatment, experimental
  Addresses   230
  Department heads   230
  Directors   230
  Financial data   230
  Patient statistical data
    230
  Personnel statistical data
    230
  Professional educational
    programs   230
  Services   230
  Telephone numbers   230
  Telex numbers   230

CANCER TREATMENT CENTERS

  RT   Cancer treatment pro-
         grams
  RT   Hospitals
  Addresses   230
  Department heads   230
  Directors   230
  Financial data   230
  Patient statistical data
    230
  Personnel statistical data

230
Professional educational
programs   230
Services   230
Telephone numbers   230
Telex numbers   230

CANCER TREATMENT PROGRAMS

RT   Cancer treatment cen-
     ters
Addresses   86
Descriptions   86
Hospital affiliations   86
Tabular data   86
Telephone numbers   86

CARBOHYDRATES

RT   Foods
RT   Nutrition
Beverages, alcoholic   54
Biochemistry
  Tabular data   94
Biosynthesis   43
Microbial composition
  Tabular data   98

CARCINOGENICITY

BT   Adverse effects
Chemical materials,
  industrial   114
Drugs   20

CARDIAC MANIFESTATIONS

RT   Cardiovascular system
Systemic diseases   205,
206

CARDIAC REHABILITATION

Nursing practice   62

CARDIAC RHYTHMS

Nursing practice   295

CARDIOPULMONARY RESUSCITATION

UF   Resuscitation
RT   Emergency care
Anesthesia   233
Techniques   27, 105, 412

CARDIOPULMONARY SURGERY

Anesthesia   233

CARDIOPULMONARY TECHNOLOGY

Indexes, literature
  Periodical literature
  315

CARDIORENAL SYSTEM

RT   Kidneys
Pathology
  Physiology   388

CARDIOVASCULAR DRUGS

Nursing practice
  Actions and uses   62
  Administration   62
  Adverse effects   62
  Dosage and administra-
  tion   62
  Elimination   62
  Indications   62
  Metabolism   62
  Warnings   62

CARDIOVASCULAR SYSTEM

NT   Arteries
NT   Heart
BT   Veins
RT   Blood
RT   Cardiac manifestations
RT   Circulation
RT   Coronary artery dis-
     eases
RT   Echocardiography
RT   Electrocardiography
RT   Hematology
RT   Hypertension
RT   Vascular diseases
 Diseases
  Diagnosis   417
  Pathophysiology   417
  Treatment, surgical
  Anatomy   417
  Anesthesia   417
  Postoperative care
  417
  Preoperative care
  417
  Techniques   417
Encyclopedias, loose-leaf

UF—Used For, BT—Broader Term, NT—Narrower Term, RT—Related Term

81, 384
Nursing practice
  Anatomy 62
  Physiology 62
Pathophysiology 331

CAS REGISTRY NUMBERS

UF Registry numbers, CAS
Chemicals 285, 370
Drugs 285, 429
Drugs, European 257

CATABOLISM   .

BT Metabolism
RT Digestion
RT Nutrition
Biochemistry 43

CATALOGS

RT Buyers' guides
RT Directories
RT Ordering information
Bacteriology
  Reference strains 39
  Type strains 39
Books, 1876-1982
  Health care 200
  Medicine 200
Books, in print
  Ordering information
    53, 265
  Publishers
    Addresses 53, 265
    Telephone numbers 53,
      265
Cultures
  Animal cell lines
    Descriptions 66
    History 66
  Packaging and shipping
    Procedures 65
    Regulations 65
  Strains, algae
    Descriptions 65
  Strains, animal viruses
    Descriptions 66
  Strains, bacteria
    Descriptions 65
  Strains, bacteriophages
    Descriptions 65
  Strains, chlamydiae
    Descriptions 66
  Strains, fungi

    Descriptions 65
  Strains, mycoviruses
    Descriptions 65
  Strains, plant viruses &
    antisera
    Descriptions 65
  Strains, protozoa
    Descriptions 65
  Strains, recombinant DNA
    vectors
    Descriptions 65
  Strains, rickettsiae
    Descriptions 66
Drug store merchandise
  Biologicals
    Prices (retail &
      wholesale) 136
  Botanicals
    Prices (retail &
      wholesale) 136
  Cosmetics
    Prices (retail &
      wholesale) 136
  Fountain products
    Prices (retail &
      wholesale) 136
  Perfumes
    Prices (retail &
      wholesale) 136
  Pharmaceuticals
    Prices (retail &
      wholesale) 136
  Stationery
    Prices (retail &
      wholesale) 136
Journals
Union lists 202
Manufacturers, drugs
  Addresses 136
  Calendars, mechandising
    136
  Drugs
    Actions and uses 136
    Adverse effects 136
    Atlases 136
    Descriptions 136
    Dosage and administra-
      tion 136
    Drug interactions 136
    Indications 136
    Packaging 136
    Warnings 136
  Identification 19
  National drug code num-
    bers 19
  Packaging 19

Prices 19
Return policies 136
Telephone numbers 136
Manufacturers, medical
devices
Addresses 267
Distributors 267
Employees, number of
267
Executives 267
FDA code numbers 267
Health risks 267
Local dealers 267
Ownership 267
Prices 267
Regulations 267
Standards 267
Telephone numbers 267
Manufacturers, surgical
instruments
Addresses 387
Illustrations 387
Ordering information
387
Telephone numbers 387
National Library of Medi-
cine
Audiovisual materials
300
Books 302
Journals 202, 219
Organizations, medical
Publications 385
Organizations, scientific
Publications 385
Reagents
Characteristics 307
Classification systems
307
Cultures 307
Potencies 307
Producers 307
Purity 307
Strains 307

CATS

BT Animals
BT Small animals
Diseases
Diagnosis 416
Etiology 416
Histopathology 416
Signs and symptoms 416
Treatment 416
Normal laboratory values

113
Physiology 416

CATTLE

BT Animals
Diseases
Autopsies 432
Control 432
Diagnosis 432
Etiology 432
Pathogenesis 432
Pathology 432
Signs and symptoms 432
Treatment 432

CAUSES OF DEATH

RT Autopsies
RT Death and dying
Medicolegal investigations
292
Statistical data 437, 443

CAVITY PREPARATION

RT Dentistry
Dentistry, operative 320

CELL BIOLOGY

BT Biology
RT Cytology
Cancer 61
Hematology 77
Pathophysiology 331
Pediatrics
Hematology 208

CELL INJURY

Pathology 329, 330

CELL LINES, ANIMAL

See Animal cell lines

CELLS

Biochemistry 43
Physiology 272, 378

CENSUS, AVERAGE DAILY

BT Statistical data
Hospitals 128, 184, 212

UF—Used For, BT—Broader Term, NT—Narrower Term, RT—Related Term

CENTRAL NERVOUS SYSTEM

See Nervous system

CERTIFICATION

RT Dental licensure
RT Examinations
RT Licensure
 Dentistry 17
 Immunology 250
 Nursing 303
 Physicians 22, 128, 424

CHAIRPERSONS

RT Administrators
RT Contact persons
RT Deans
RT Department heads
RT Directors
RT Officials
 University programs
  Allied health sciences
  341
  Biological sciences 341
  Dentistry 341
  Medicine 341
  Nursing 341
  Pharmacy 341
  Public health 341
  Veterinary medicine 341

CHARGES

RT Fees
RT Prices
 Diseases
  Hospitals 332

CHEMICAL COMPOUNDS

RT Chemicals
 Chemical names
  Synonyms 342
 Pharmacological names
  Synonyms 342
 Trade names
  Synonyms 342

CHEMICAL CONSTANTS

 Biology
  Tabular data 48

CHEMICAL CONSTITUENTS

Blood 52
Body fluids
 Adverse effects 105
Plants, medicinal 247

CHEMICAL FORMULATIONS

Brand names 68
Chemical manufacturers 68
Trademarks 68

CHEMICAL HAZARDS

RT Chemical materials, in-
    dustrial
RT Occupational health
Occupational diseases
 Adverse effects 319
 Diagnostic tests 319
 Permissible exposure
 limits 319
 Personnel protective
 measures 319
 Routes of entry 319

CHEMICAL MANUFACTURERS

See Manufacturers, chemi-
 cals

CHEMICAL MATERIALS, INDUSTRI-
AL

RT Chemical hazards
RT Chemicals
RT Commercial products,
    chemicals
 Air pollution
  Control 114
  Hazards 114
 Carcinogenicity 114
 Descriptions 114
 Explosion data 114
 Fires
  Control 114
  Hazards 114
 Flammability data 114
 Hazard data 114
 Noise pollution
  Control 114
  Hazards 114
 Occupational health 114
 Physical constants 114
 Radiation pollution
  Control 114
  Hazards 114

Regulations 114
Solid wastes
  Control   114
  Hazards   114
Synonyms 114
Toxicology
  Test animals
    Quantity of exposure
    114
    Route of exposure   114
Ventilation procedures
114
Waste disposal 114

CHEMICAL NAMES

UF Names, chemical
Chemical compounds
  Synonyms   342
Drugs   18, 429
  Synonyms   342
Drugs, nonprescription
349
Drugs, prescription 348
Pesticides
  Synonyms   342

CHEMICALS

NT Chemicals, European
NT Commercial products,
    chemicals
NT Drugs
NT Insecticides
NT Pesticides
NT Solvents
RT Chemical compounds
RT Chemical materials,
    industrial
RT Manufacturers, chemi-
    cals
Actions and uses   285
Composition 285
CAS registry numbers   285,
370
Molecular formulas   285,
370
Molecular weights   285,
370
Poisoning
  Diagnosis   193, 351
  Prevention   193
  Prognosis   193
  Signs and symptoms 193,
  351
  Treatment   193

Structural formulas   285
Synonyms   285, 370
Tabular data
  Handbooks   95
Teratogenic agents
  Abstracts, literature
  64
  Indexes, literature   64
Toxicology 285
  Bibliographies, annotat-
  ed   370
  Regulations   370
  Standards   370
  Trademarks   285

CHEMICALS, EUROPEAN

BT Chemicals
NT Drugs, British
NT Drugs, European
RT Manufacturers, drugs,
    European
Analysis
  Techniques   155
Assays   155
Characteristics   155
Identification   155
Labelling   155
Molecular formulas   155
Potencies   155
Reagents   155
Storage 155
Structural formulas   155
Tests   155

CHEMISTRY

NT Biochemistry
RT Elements
RT Laboratory sciences,
    clinical
RT Reagents
CRC handbooks
  Indexes   93
Drugs   20, 175
Glossaries   95
Graduate schools
  Ratings   176
Heavy metals
  Toxicology   175
Pharmaceutical practice
371
Poisoning
  Animals, marine   352
Undergraduate schools
  Ratings   177

UF–Used For, BT–Broader Term, NT–Narrower Term, RT–Related Term

CHEMOPROPHYLAXIS

  RT Immunizations
  RT Prevention
   Travelers
     Tropical medicine   215

CHEST

  See Thorax

CHEST ROENTGEN SCREENING

  BT Diagnosis, radiologic
   Respiratory system   117

CHILD DEVELOPMENT

  BT Growth and development
   Expected tasks   296
   Suggested tasks   296

CHILD PSYCHIATRY

  BT Psychiatry
  RT Mental illness
   Diseases
     Diagnosis   89
     Epidemiology   89
     Etiology   89
     Signs and symptoms   89
     Treatment   89

CHILDBIRTH

  UF Birth
  UF Delivery
  UF Labor
  NT Home birth
  RT Antepartal care
  RT Birth fractures
  RT Gynecology
  RT Midwives, number of
  RT Obstetrics
  RT Postpartum period
  RT Pregnancy
  RT Puerperium
   Gynecology   106
   Obstetrics   191
     Complications   441
     Physiology   441
     Techniques   441
   Patient education   21
   Pregnancy   318
     Nursing practice   258
     Obstetrics   191

  Treatment, surgical
   Obstetrics   321

CHILDREN, CARE OF

  See Pediatrics

CHLAMYDIAE

  See Strains, Chlamydiae

CHOKING

  BT Accidents
  RT Emergency care
   Treatment   105, 136

CHOLESTEROL CONTENT

  RT Nutrition
   Foods   54, 187, 245

CHROMATOGRAPHY

   Biochemistry
     Tabular data   94

CHROMOSOMAL ANOMALIES

  UF Anomalies, chromosomal
  RT Birth defects
  RT Teratology
   Abstracts, literature   69
   Atlases   69
   Etiology   69
   Genetics   270
   Natural history   69
   Signs and symptoms   69
   Tabular data   69

CIGARETTE SMOKING

  See Smoking (tobacco)

CIRCULATION

  RT Cardiovascular system
  RT Hematology
   Biology
     Tabular data   48
   Physiology   40, 272, 378

CLASSIFICATION SYSTEMS

  RT Nomenclature
  RT Taxonomy

RT   Terminology
Animals
  Biology 209
Arthropods
  Parasitology 83
Bacteria 39
  Microbiology 251
Birth defects 339
Books
  Medicine 301
Burns
  Nursing practice 144
Cancer 60
  Morphology 229
Chemicals, toxicology 229
Dermatology 256
Diagnosis 229
Diseases 229, 398
  Dermatology 116
  Emergency care 143
  Encyclopedias, loose-
    leaf 81
  Gynecology 191
  Ophthalmology 171
  Psychiatry 89
Dislocations
  Orthopedics 165
Drugs 298
  Nursing practice 312
  Toxicology 229
Enzymes 154
Fractures
  Orthopedics 165
Helminths
  Parasitology 83
Injuries 229
  Orthopedics 165
Mental illness 118
Nervous system
  Nursing practice 63
Pathology
  Diseases 398
  Etiology 398
  Morphology 398
  Occupations 398
  Physiology 398
  Techniques 398
  Topography 398
Plants
  Biology 209
  Poisoning 353
Plastic surgery 369
Procedures
  Anesthesiology 347
  Diagnosis, radiologic
    347

Laboratory techniques
  347
Medicine 347
Pathology 347
Treatment, surgical 347
Protozoa
  Parasitology 83
Reagents 307
Services
  Anesthesiology 347
  Diagnosis, radiologic
    347
  Laboratory medicine 347
  Medicine 347
  Pathology 347
  Treatment, surgical 347
Trauma
  Emergency care 143
Treatment, surgical 229
Viruses
  Animals 146

CLEARINGHOUSES, HEALTH

  Nursing 303

CLINICAL PHARMACOLOGY

  BT   Pharmacology
  Handbooks
    Drug prescribing
      Breast feeding 188
      Dietary considerations
        188
      Diseases, drug induced
        188
      Drug interactions 188
      Geriatric drug use
        188
      Immunization schedules
        188
      Nomograms 188
      Parenteral nutrition
        188
      Pharmacogenetics 188

CLINICS

  RT   Health care services
  RT   Hospitals
    Directories 203

COAGULATION FACTORS

  RT   Hematology
    Pediatrics 208

UF-Used For, BT-Broader Term, NT-Narrower Term, RT-Related Term

COLLEGES

See Education for specific
types

COLON

BT   Alimentary tract
BT   Gastrointestinal system
Diseases
Signs and symptoms   394
Treatment, surgical
393, 394

COMA

Differential diagnosis
244

COMBINING FORMS

NT   Greek combining forms
NT   Latin combining forms
RT   Terminology
Dictionaries   145

COMMERCIAL PRODUCTS, CHEMI-
CALS

BT   Chemicals
RT   Chemical materials,
industrial
RT   Cosmetics
RT   Drug store merchandise
RT   Household products
RT   Perfumes
Formulas   85
Ingredients   85
Manufacturers
Addresses   85
Telephone numbers   85
Poisoning
Emergency care   85
Signs and symptoms   85
Treatment   85
Toxicity ratings   85
Toxicology
Emergency care   85
Signs and symptoms   85
Treatment   85
Trade names   85

COMMUNICABLE DISEASES

UF   Infectious diseases
BT   Diseases

NT   Nosocomial infections
NT   Sexually transmitted
diseases
RT   Fungi
RT   Infection control
RT   Mycology
RT   Public health
RT   Rickettsiae
RT   Vaccines
RT   Viruses
Communicability periods
91, 296
Complications
Public health   259
Control 91, 223
Public health   259
Diagnosis   91, 223, 354,
355
Public health   259
Diagnosis, laboratory
223, 354
Drugs (treatment modality)
Actions and uses   354,
355
Adverse effects   355
Availability   355
Dosage and administra-
tion   354, 355
Pharmacology   355
Encyclopedias, loose-leaf
384
Epidemiology   223, 354,
355
Public health   259
Etiology   223
Public health   259
History
Public health   259
Immunizations   37
Adverse effects   354
Indications   354
Schedules   354
Warnings   354
Immunology
Public health   259
Immunopathology   223
Incubation periods   91,
296
Infectious agents   91
Occurrence   91
Public health   259
Pathogenesis   223, 355
Pathology   223
Physiology   388
Public health   259
Pediatrics

Communicability periods
296
Complications 224, 296
Control 296
Diagnosis 224, 373
Differential diagnosis
224
Epidemiology 224
Etiology 224, 373
Immunizations 224, 373
Incubation periods 296
Nursing practice 296
Pathogenesis 224
Pathology 224
Prognosis 224
Signs and symptoms 224,
296
Sources 296
Transmission 296
Treatment 224, 296, 373
Prevention 91, 223, 355
Public health 259
Prognosis 223, 355
Public health
Complications 259
Control 259
Diagnosis 259
Epidemiology 259
Etiology 259
History 259
Immunology 259
Occurrence 259
Pathology 259
Prevention 259
Signs and symptoms 259
Transmission 259
Treatment 259
Reservoir 91
Resistance 91
Signs and symptoms 223,
296, 354, 355
Public health 259
Susceptibility 91
Transmission 91, 296
Public health 259
Treatment 91, 223, 354,
355
Public health 259
Treatment, surgical 360
Diagnosis 395
Epidemiology 395
Etiology 395
Handbooks 110
Microbiology 395
Pathogenesis 395
Prognosis 395

Signs and symptoms 395
Treatment 395
Wound infections 395
Tropical medicine
Control 215
Diagnosis 215
Distribution 215
Etiology 215
History 215
Pathogenesis 215
Pathophysiology 215
Prevention 215
Prognosis 215
Signs and symptoms 215
Transmission 215
Treatment 215

COMMUNITY MENTAL HEALTH CEN-
TERS

RT Mental illness
Directories 203

COMPANIES

See Manufacturers

COMPATIBILITY

Drugs, injectable 194

COMPLEMENT SYSTEM

Immunology 37, 250

COMPLICATIONS

RT Adverse effects
Anesthesia 233
Birth defects 49
Cancer 60
Childbirth
Obstetrics 441
Communicable diseases
Public health 259
Diseases
Encyclopedias, loose-
leaf 81
Gastrointestinal system
169
Genitourinary system
172
Gynecology 191
Handbooks 105
Heart 206
Immunology 37

Pediatrics   339
Treatment, surgical
   Handbooks   110
Dislocations   165
Drugs (treatment modality)
   Mental illness   189
Food poisoning   259
Fractures   165
Injuries   165
Mental illness   118
Nosocomial infections   259
Pediatrics
   Anesthesia   29
   Infections, postopera-
      tive   397
   Communicable diseases
      224, 296
Postoperative care   255
Pregnancy   318
   Biochemistry   266
   Nursing practice   258
   Obstetrics   191, 441
   Physiology   266
   Signs and symptoms   266
   Treatment   266
Preoperative care
   Treatment, surgical   255
Sexually transmitted dis-
   eases   259
Shock treatment
   Nursing practice   144
Treatment, surgical
   Diseases
      Gynecology   401
   Handbooks   110
   Urology   107

COMPUTED TOMOGRAPHY

BT   Diagnosis, radiologic
Encyclopedias, loose-leaf
   81
   Nervous system   82

COMPUTERS

RT   Data bases
Practice management   406

CONCEPTION

RT   Gynecology
RT   Pregnancy
RT   Reproduction
Endocrine system
   Gynecology   76

CONFERENCES

See Meetings, future
See Meetings, past

CONGENITAL ANOMALIES

See Birth defects

CONGRESSIONAL SUBCOMMITTEES

RT   Senators and represen-
      tatives
Health care
   Addresses   299
   Birth dates   299
   Birth places   299
   Career biographies   299
   Health staff aides   299
   Photographs   299
   Telephone numbers   299

CONNECTIVE TISSUE

RT   Histology
Pathophysiology   331

CONSTIPATION

Differential diagnosis
   244

CONSTITUTION

U.S. Pharmacopeial Convention   426

CONSULTANTS

Health care
   Directories   381
      Addresses   261
      Services   261
      Telephone numbers   261

CONSUMER HEALTH

See Patient education

CONTACT PERSONS

RT   Administrators
RT   Chairpersons
RT   Deans
RT   Department heads
RT   Directors

RT   Executives
RT   Officials
Boards of pharmacy, state
  136
Certifying boards
  Dental licensure 17
Health care services
  Pediatrics 297
Manufacturers, drugs 348,
  349
Manufacturers, health care
  products, Canada 58
Meetings, future 386, 444
Mental health services
  Pediatrics 297
Organizations, dental 17
Organizations, pharmaceu-
  tical 136
Runaway youth centers 297
Senators and representa-
  tives 299

CONTENTS, TABLES OF

See Tables of contents

CONTINUING EDUCATION

Nursing 317

CONTRACEPTION

UF   Birth control
UF   Family planning
NT   Sterilization
Directories 381
Gynecology 311
Obstetrics 441
Patient education 21
Sexuality
  Nursing practice 214
  Psychological aspects
    89
  Techniques 89

CONTRAINDICATIONS

See Warnings

CONTROL MECHANISMS

Metabolism 288

CONVENTIONS

See Meetings, future

See Meetings, past

CONVERSION TABLES

Pediatrics 195
Weights and measures 246

CONVULSIONS

Differential diagnosis
  244

COPY EDITING

RT   Style manuals
RT   Writing, medical
Manuals 249

CORE COLLECTIONS

Reference books
  Indexes, thesauri 162

CORONARY ARTERY DISEASES

BT   Diseases
RT   Cardiovascular system
RT   Heart
Nursing practice
  Diagnosis 62
  Pathophysiology 62
  Patient assessment 62
  Treatment 62

CORONERS

NT   Physicians
RT   Death and dying
Directories 381

COSMETICS

BT   Drug store merchandise
RT   Commercial products,
       chemicals
RT   Household products
RT   Perfumes
Encyclopedias
  Chemical composition
    149
  Commercially available
    forms 149
  Natural ingredients 149
  Pharmacology 149
  Physical descriptions
    149

UF-Used For, BT-Broader Term, NT-Narrower Term, RT-Related Term

Plant sources   149
Preparation methods   149
Synonyms   149
Poisoning
   Diagnosis   193, 351
   Prevention   193
   Prognosis   193
   Signs and symptoms   193,
   351
   Treatment   193, 351
Prices (retail & whole-
sale)
   Catalogs   136

COST

See Prices

COUGH

Differential diagnosis
244

COUNCIL ON DENTAL THERAPEU-
TICS

BT   Organizations, dental
   Members   5
   Product acceptance cri-
      teria   5

COUNSELING SERVICES

BT   Mental health services
NT   Family counseling
NT   Sex counseling
RT   Mental illness
   Directories   203

COURTROOM EVIDENCE

RT   Forensic science
RT   Law
   Presentation techniques
      Forensic psychiatry   292
      Medicolegal investiga-
         tions   292

CRC HANDBOOKS

BT   Handbooks
RT   Tabular data
   Indexes
      Analytical toxicology
      93
      Biochemistry   93

Chemistry   93
Engineering
   Biology   93
   Medicine   93
Flavor ingredients   93
Food additives   93
Foods   93
Laboratory animal
   science   93
Laboratory safety   93
Laboratory science,
   clinical   93
Mathematics   93
Microbiology   93
Molecular biology   93
Nutrition   93
Physics   93
Probability   93
Radioactive nuclides   93
Scientific tables   93
Statistical data   93

CRIME

See Forensic science

CRITICAL CARE

UF   Life support
RT   Accidents
RT   Critical care unit per-
      sonnel
RT   Emergency care
RT   High risk patients
RT   Injuries
RT   Intensive care
   Encyclopedias, loose-leaf
   81
   Nursing practice
      Anatomy   100
      Burns   100
      Cardiac rhythms   295
      Critical care units   295
      Diabetes   100
      Diseases
         Diagnosis   100
         Pathophysiology   100
         Treatment   100
      Drug overdose   100
      Drugs (treatment modal-
      ity)
         Adverse effects   295
         Dosage and administra-
            tion   295
         Indications   295
         Routes of administra-

tion 295
Electrocardiograms
  Interpretations 295
Gastrointestinal bleed-
  ing 100
Hepatic failure 100
History and physical ex-
  amination
  Techniques 295
Holistic approach 100
Infection control 295
Life support
  Techniques 295
Physiology 100
Poisoning 100

CRITICAL CARE UNIT PERSONNEL

  RT Critical care
  Nursing practice
    Job burnout 100
    Job training 100
    Legal aspects 100
    Stress 100

CROSS RESISTANCE

  Treatment, chemical
    Cancer 79

CROSS-SENSITIVITY

  RT Drug interactions
  Drugs 428
    Patient education 427

CULTURE AND ISOLATION

  RT Culture media
  RT Cultures
  Bacteriology
    Microbiology 251
  Fungi
    Microbiology 251
  Parasitology
    Microbiology 251
  Rickettsiae
    Microbiology 251
  Spirochetes
    Microbiology 251
  Viruses
    Microbiology 251

CULTURE MEDIA

  RT Culture and isolation

  RT Cultures
  Biology
    Tabular data 48
  Microbiology
    Formulas 35
    Procedures 35

CULTURES

  RT Culture and isolation
  RT Culture media
  Catalogs
    Animal cell lines
      Descriptions 66
      History 66
    Packaging and shipping
      Procedures 65
      Regulations 65
    Reagents
      Ordering information
      307
    Strains, algae
      Descriptions 65
    Strains, animal viruses
      Descriptions 66
    Strains, bacteria
      Descriptions 65
    Strains, bacteriophages
      Descriptions 65
    Strains, chlamydiae
      Descriptions 66
    Strains, fungi
      Descriptions 65
    Strains, mycoviruses
      Descriptions 65
    Strains, plant viruses &
      antisera
      Descriptions 65
    Strains, protozoa
      Descriptions 65
    Strains, recombinant DNA
      vectors
      Descriptions 65
    Strains, rickettsiae
      Descriptions 66

CURRICULA

  Dental schools
    Directories 10, 36
  Medical schools
    Directories 1, 36, 275

CYANOSIS

  Differential diagnosis

244

CYTOGENETICS

  BT   Genetics
  RT   Cytology
  Gynecology   311, 318

CYTOLOGY

  BT   Biology
  RT   Cell biology
  RT   Cytogenetics
  Biology
    Tabular data   48
  Hematology   77

CYTOPATHOLOGY

  BT   Pathology
  Gynecology   310
  Obstetrics   310

DATA BASE ACCESS

  RT   Healthline
  RT   Medline
  RT   Popline
  Libraries, medical
    Directories   125

DATA BASES

  RT   Computers
  NT   Healthline
  NT   Medline
  NT   Popline
  Toxicology
    Information sources   225

DATES

  NT   Birth dates
  Applied sciences
    Meetings, past   221
  Medicine
    Meetings, future   386,
    444
    Meetings, past   127,
    221
  Sciences
    Meetings, future   386
    Meetings, past   127, 221

DEAF SERVICES

  BT   Handicapped services
  RT   Sign language
  Directories   203

DEANS

  RT   Administrators
  RT   Chairpersons
  RT   Contact persons
  RT   Department heads
  RT   Directors
  RT   Officials
  Allied health sciences
    schools   261
  Medical schools   261
  Public health schools
    46

DEATH AND DYING

  RT   Asphyxial deaths
  RT   Autopsies
  RT   Causes of death
  RT   Coroners
  RT   Dying declarations
  RT   Dying patients
  RT   Mortality
  RT   Sudden infant death
       syndrome centers
  RT   Suicides
  RT   Terminal care
  RT   Time of death
  RT   Trauma deaths
  RT   Vital statistics
  Aged   72
  Anatomical donations   389
  Bereavement counseling
    389
  Estate planning   389
  Euthanasia   389
  Funeral industry
    Licensing requirements
    389
  Funeral practices   389
  Funeral service schools
    Addresses   389
    Programs offered   389
    Telephone numbers   389
  Hospice care   389
  Information sources   389
  Legal aspects   389
  Nursing practice   241
  Patient education   21
  Patient rights   389
  Pediatrics
    Medicolegal investiga-

tions 292
Statistical data 389
Wills 389

DEATH INVESTIGATIONS

Forensic science 292

DEATH RATE

See Mortality

DECISION TREES

RT Diagnosis
Differential diagnosis
Mental illness 118
Respiratory system 117

DEFICIENCIES, NUTRITIONAL

See Nutritional deficien-
cies

DEHYDRATION

Differential diagnosis
244

DELEGATE ROSTER

Association of Cancer
Centers 86

DELIVERY

See Childbirth

DENTAL CARE, HOSPITAL

RT Dentistry
RT Dentistry, operative
American Dental Associa-
tion
Standards 210
Diagnosis 210
Emergency dental care 210
Infection control 210
Laboratory service 210
Medical records 210
Operating room procedures
210
Patient admission 210
Pediatric patients 210

DENTAL LICENSURE

BT Licensure
RT Certification
Certifying boards
Addresses 17
Contact persons 17
Statistical data 17

DENTAL SCHOOLS

UF Education, dental
BT University programs
RT Dentistry
Academic calendars 10
Addresses 10, 36, 216,
341
Admission requirements
10, 36
Admission statistics 36
Chairpersons 341
Curricula 10, 36
Degrees awarded 10
Expenses 10, 36
Facilities 36
Faculty, number of 341
Financial aid 10, 36
Programs offered 341
Ratings 176
Selection criteria 10
Students, number of 341
Telephone numbers 341
University community 341

DENTISTRY

NT Forensic dentistry
RT Cavity preparation
RT Dental care, hospital
RT Dental schools
RT Mouth
RT Oral diseases
RT Oral manifestations
RT Organizations, dental
RT Pulp protection
Abbreviations 3, 216
Acronyms 216
Aged 72
Dictionaries 101, 216
Directories
Bibliographies 124
Diseases
Diagnosis
Instruments 345
Techniques 345
Epidemiology 259
Prevention 5, 259
Drugs (treatment modality)

UF-Used For, BT-Broader Term, NT-Narrower Term, RT-Related Term

Actions and uses 5
Adverse effects 5
Chemical descriptions 5
Distributors 5
Trade names 5
Warnings 5
Educational planning 10
Indexes, literature 218
Initialisms 216
Pediatrics
  Anesthesia 29
Research programs
  Addresses 376
  Cable addresses 376
  Officials 376
  Research activities 376
  Staff, number of 376
  Telephone numbers 376
  Telex numbers 376
  TWX numbers 376
Sign language 276
Thesauri 262
Trademarks 216

DENTISTRY, OPERATIVE

RT   Dental care, hospital
RT   Dentistry
RT   Maxilla
Cavity preparation 320
Diagnosis 320
Pulp protection 320
Restorations 320
Treatment planning 320

DENTISTS

See American Dental Association

DEPARTMENT HEADS

RT   Administrators
RT   Chairpersons
RT   Contact persons
RT   Deans
RT   Directors
RT   Officials
Cancer research institutes
  230
Cancer treatment centers
  230
Hospitals 58
Hospitals, United Kingdom
  268
Medical schools, United

Kingdom 268

DERMATOLOGY

UF   Skin
UF   Skin diseases
RT   Skin grafting
RT   Skin manifestations
Anatomy 116
Biology 116
Diseases
  Atlases 116, 256
  Classification systems
    116, 256
  Diagnosis 26, 116, 256
  Diagnosis, laboratory
    26, 256
  Differential diagnosis
    26, 256
  Epidemiology 26, 116
  Etiology 26, 256
  Histopathology 26
  Natural histories 256
  Pathogenesis 26, 116
  Pathology 116
  Pathophysiology 26,
    116, 331
  Prevention 116
  Prognosis 116
  Signs and symptoms 26,
    116, 256
  Treatment 26, 116, 256
Encyclopedias, loose-leaf
  81, 384
Growth and development
  116
Hormones 405
Systemic diseases
  Skin manifestations 116

DEVELOPMENT

See Growth and development

DIABETES

BT   Diseases
RT   Endocrine system
Emergency care 100
Immunizations 37

DIAGNOSIS

UF   Assessment
NT   Diagnosis, immunologic
NT   Diagnosis, laboratory

NT   Diagnosis, radiologic
NT   Diagnosis, ultrasound
NT   Differential diagnosis
NT   Echocardiography
NT   Electroencephalography
NT   Serodiagnosis
RT   Decision trees
RT   History and physical
     examination
Abdomen   4
Acid-base disturbances
 236
Adrenals   57
Aged   72
Allergy   12
Ambulatory medicine   358
Animals   131
Arthropods
  Parasitology   83
Athletic injuries   419
Bile ducts   132, 133
Birth defects   49
Birth fractures   115
Bites and stings   193, 351
Blood vessels   205
Cancer   7, 60, 61
Cardiovascular system   417
Cats
  Veterinary medicine   416
Cattle
  Veterinary medicine   432
Child psychiatry   89
Communicable diseases   91,
 223, 354, 355, 395
  Public health   259
  Tropical medicine   215
Coronary artery diseases
  Nursing practice   62
Critical care
  Nursing practice   100
Dentistry   210, 345
Dentistry, operative   320
Dermatology   26, 116, 256
Disability, physical   237
Dislocations   165
  Atlases   115
Dogs
  Veterinary medicine
   416
Drug abuse
  Psychiatry   89
Electrolyte disturbances
 74, 236, 372, 392
Emergency care   142, 143,
 253, 290, 350
Encyclopedias   196

Encyclopedias, loose-leaf
 81
Endocrine system   153, 405
  Gynecology   76
Fluid disturbances   74,
 236
Fracture-dislocations
  Atlases   115
Fractures   165
  Atlases   115
Gallbladder   132, 133
Gastrointestinal system
 75, 168, 169
Genetics   270, 287
Genitourinary system   172
Genitourinary system, fe-
 male   185
Gynecology   106, 311, 318
Handbooks   104, 105, 253,
 286, 350
  Pediatrics   439
Heart   173, 205, 206
Helminths
  Parasitology   83
Hematology   77, 207
Horses
  Veterinary medicine   432
Injuries
  Orthopedics   165
Internal medicine   67,
 196, 281, 288, 356, 406
Kidneys   236, 372, 392
Liver   132, 133
Lungs   173
Mental illness   89, 291
Metabolism   288
Nervous system   82, 92,
 306, 359, 408
  Nursing practice   63
Newborns   382
Nosocomial infections   259
Nursing practice   242, 294
Nutritional deficiencies
  Tropical medicine   215
Ophthalmology   171, 322,
 323
Oral manifestations
  Systemic diseases   399
Original articles
  Bibliographies   152
Orthopedics   254, 326
Otolaryngology   328, 411
Parasitology   83, 168
Patient education   21
Pediatrics   108, 304, 339
  Communicable diseases

UF-Used For, BT-Broader Term, NT-Narrower Term, RT-Related Term

224, 373
Emergency care   252
Gastrointestinal system
335
Handbooks   192, 195, 439
Nursing practice   88
Ophthalmology   336
Orthopedics   337
Speech disorders   411
Pigs
Veterinary medicine   432
Poisoning
Chemicals   193, 351
Cosmetics   193, 351
Drugs   193, 351
Fish   215
Foods   168, 193, 259
Household products   351
Industrial hazards   351
Insecticides   351
Plants   193, 351
Tropical medicine   215
Snakebites
Tropical medicine   215
Veterinary medicine
Small animals   113
Pregnancy
Animals   146
Nursing practice   258
Obstetrics   191
Protozoa
Parasitology   83
Psychiatry   89, 291
Respiratory system   365,
366, 413
Rheumatology   31, 84, 414
Sexually transmitted dis-
eases
Public health   259
Sheep
Veterinary medicine   432
Small animals
Veterinary medicine   113
Subluxations
Atlases   115
Techniques
Atlases   70
Thorax   173, 417
Toxicology
Heavy metals   175
Trauma   143
Nursing practice 144
Urology   57

DIAGNOSIS, IMMUNOLOGIC

BT   Diagnosis
RT   Immunology
Arthropods
Parasitology   83
Diseases   37
Helminths
Parasitology   83
Protozoa
Parasitology   83

DIAGNOSIS, LABORATORY

UF   Laboratory diagnosis
BT   Diagnosis
RT   Laboratories
RT   Laboratory techniques
Acid-base disturbances
Nursing practice   314
Allergy   250
Bacteriology
Media formulas   179
Reagents   179
Staining techniques   179
Stains formulas   179
Tests   179
Body fluid disturbances
Nursing practice   314
Classification systems
347
Communicable diseases
223, 354
Dermatology   26, 256
Electrolyte disturbances
Nursing practice   314
Encyclopedias, loose-leaf
81
Endocrine system
Gynecology   76
Hematology
Atlases   240
Calculations   207
Equipment   207
Interpretations   207
Interpretations of tests
179
Laboratory techniques
179
Normal laboratory values
240
Principles   207
Purpose   207
Reagents   207, 240
Reagents sources   207
Techniques   207, 240
Immunology
Immunodeficiency dis-

eases   250
Interpretations of tests
179
Laboratory techniques
179
Procedures   37
Mycology
Interpretations of tests
179
Laboratory techniques
179
Nursing practice
Abbreviations   239
Interferences   239
Normal ranges   239
Nursing implications   239
Techniques   239
Occupational diseases
Pesticides   319
Parasitology
Interpretations of tests
179
Laboratory techniques
179
Tests
Atlases   70
Classification systems
229
Indications   231
Pediatrics   232
Interferences   135, 231,
428
Pediatrics   232
Interpretations   30, 80,
179, 231, 418
Pediatrics   232
Techniques   80, 179, 418

DIAGNOSIS, RADIOLOGIC

UF   Radiologic diagnosis
BT   Diagnosis
NT   Chest roentgen screen-
ing
NT   Computed tomography
NT   Neuroradiography
RT   Nuclear medicine
RT   Radioactive nuclides
RT   Radiographic anatomy
RT   Radioisotopes
RT   Radiologic technology
Diseases   38, 174, 334
Emergency care   367
Malnutrition   293
Metabolism   368
Nervous system   82

Orthopedics   327
Pediatrics   338
Rheumatology   31
Human body parts
Anatomy   174
History   174
Physiology   174
Techniques   174
Injuries
Emergency care   367
Postoperative care
Treatment, surgical   396
Preoperative care
Treatment, surgical   396
Procedures
Classification systems
347
Services
Classification systems
347
Syndromes   368
Treatment, surgical   396

DIAGNOSIS, ULTRASOUND

BT   Diagnosis
RT   Ultrasonography
Diseases   404

DIAGNOSTIC SERVICES

Directories   203

DIARRHEA

Differential diagnosis
244

DICTIONARIES

NT   Dictionaries, illustra-
ted
NT   Dictionaries, inverted
NT   Dictionaries, reversed
NT   English-Spanish glossa-
ries
RT   Encyclopedias
RT   Glossaries
RT   Keywords
RT   Polyglots
RT   Synonyms
RT   Terminology
Allied health sciences
52, 145
Biology   209
Combining forms

UF-Used For, BT-Broader Term, NT-Narrower Term, RT-Related Term

Medical terminology   145
Dentistry   101, 216
Diseases
  Etiology   217
  Inheritance   217
  Metabolism   217
  Original articles
    Bibliographies   217
  Pathology   217
  Signs and symptoms   50,
    217
  Synonyms   217
  Treatment   50
Drugs
  Actions and uses   50
Internal medicine   67
Keywords
  Medicine   235, 377
Management
  Health sciences   120
Medicine   50, 52, 134,
  145, 391, 400
Nursing   145, 246, 296
Orthopedics   326
  Abbreviations   254
  Amputation   326
  Anatomy   254
  Diagnostic techniques
    254
  Diseases   254
    Diagnosis   326
    Etiology   326
    Pathology   326
    Signs and symptoms
      326
    Treatment   326
  Dislocations   254
  Fractures   254
  Physical medicine   254
  Positions, anatomical
    254
  Skin grafting   326
  Tests   254
  Treatment   254
Psychiatry   364
Quotations
  Medicine   161
Syndromes
  Etiology   217
  Inheritance   217
  Metabolism   217
  Original articles
    Bibliographies   217
  Pathology   217
  Signs and symptoms   217
  Synonyms   217

Veterinary medicine
  Diseases
    Signs and symptoms
      51
  Drugs
    Actions and uses   51

DICTIONARIES, ILLUSTRATED

  BT   Dictionaries
  Medicine   283

DICTIONARIES, INVERTED

  BT   Dictionaries
  Terminology, medical   235

DICTIONARIES, REVERSED

  BT   Dictionaries
  Medicine   377

DIETETICS, CLINICAL

  RT   Nutrition
  Handbooks   187

DIETS, MODIFIED

  RT   Foods
  RT   Nutrition
  Adverse effects   187
  Food choice recommenda-
    tions   187
  Indications   187
  Patient education   227
  Purposes   187

DIFFERENTIAL DIAGNOSIS

  BT   Diagnosis
  RT   Signs and symptoms
  Anatomical pathology
    Nervous system   359
  Anemia
    Diseases   244
  Bleeding
    Diseases   244
  Coma
    Diseases   244
  Communicable diseases
    Pediatrics   224
  Constipation
    Diseases   244
  Convulsions
    Diseases   244

Cough
  Diseases   244
Cyanosis
  Diseases   244
Decision trees
  Respiratory system   117
Dehydration
  Diseases   244
Diarrhea
  Diseases   244
Diseases   38, 122, 166
  Dermatology   26, 256
  Emergency care   142
    Pediatrics   412
  Genetics   270
  Gynecology   191
  Handbooks   104, 105
  Hematology   77
  Immunology   37
  Metabolism   368
  Nervous system   92
  Pediatrics   108, 192
  Rheumatology   31, 84,
  414
Dizziness
  Diseases   244
Dyspnea
  Diseases   244
Edema
  Diseases   244
Fatigue
  Diseases   244
Fever
  Diseases   244
Headache
  Diseases   244
Hypertension
  Diseases   244
Jaundice
  Diseases   244
Malnutrition
  Diseases   244
Mental illness
  Decision trees   118
Nausea
  Diseases   244
Nervousness
  Diseases   244
Obesity
  Diseases   244
Pain
  Diseases   244
  Nursing practice   63
Pallor
  Diseases   244
Pruritus

  Diseases   244
Skin color
  Diseases   244
Syncope
  Diseases   244
Syndromes   368
Vertigo
  Diseases   244

DIGESTION

  RT   Catabolism
  RT   Metabolism
  RT   Pancreas
  Biology
    Tabular data   48
  Physiology   40, 272

DIRECTORIES

  RT   Addresses
  RT   Biographies
  RT   Buyers' guides
  RT   Catalogs
  RT   Information sources
  RT   Telephone numbers
  Allied health sciences
  schools
    Academic calendars   13
    Accreditation   13
    Addresses   13, 261, 341
    Admission requirements
    13
    Affiliates   13
    Certificates awarded   13
    Chairpersons   341
    Deans   261
    Degrees awarded   13
    Faculty, number of   341
    Financial aid   13
    Programs offered   341
    Students, number of   341
    Telephone numbers   13,
    261, 341
    Tuition   13, 341
    University community
    341
  American College of Physicians
    Members
      Addresses   45
      Awards   45
      Birth dates   45
      Birth places   45
      Educational back-
      grounds   45

UF—Used For, BT—Broader Term, NT—Narrower Term, RT—Related Term

Marriage dates 45
Professional activi-
  ties 45
Professional certifi-
  cations 45
Specialties 45
Spouses 45
Telephone numbers 45
Officials 45
American College of Sur-
geons
Members
  Addresses 16
  Birth dates 16
  Dates of membership
    16
  Educational back-
    grounds 16
  Professional certifi-
    cations 16
  Professional member-
    ships 16
  Specialties 16
American Dental Associa-
tion
Members
  Addresses 17
  Birth dates 17
  Educational back-
    grounds 17
  Membership status 17
Officials
  Addresses 17
American Hospital Associa-
tion
Awards 184
Members
  Addresses 184
Officials 184
American Medical Association
Committee members
  Addresses 14
  Telephone numbers 14
Officials
  Addresses 14
  Telephone numbers 14
Staff members
  Addresses 14
  Telephone numbers 14
Trustees
  Addresses 14
  Telephone numbers 14
American Psychiatry Asso-
ciation
Members
  Addresses 44

Birth dates 44
Certification 44
Educational back-
  grounds 44
Employment status 44
Hospital affiliations
  44
Professional activi-
  ties 44
Professional member-
  ships 44
Publications 44
Telephone numbers 44
Officials 44
American Public Health As-
sociation
Members
  Addresses 46
  Awards 46
  Birth dates 46
  Birth places 46
  Educational back-
    grounds 46
  Professional certifi-
    cations 46
  Professional experi-
    ence 46
  Telephone numbers 46
Archives
Addresses 129
Directors 129
Founding dates 129
Holdings
  Statistical data 129
Networks and consortia
  129
Publications 129
Services 129
Special collections 129
Staff names 129
Staff, number of 129
Subjects 129
Telephone numbers 129
Association of American
Medical Colleges
Activities 2
Awards 2
Members 2
Officials 2
Bibliographies
Allied health sciences
  Addresses 124
  Circulations 124
  Editors 124
  Frequencies 124
  Prices 124

Scopes   124
  Telephone numbers   124
Dentistry
  Addresses   124
  Circulations   124
  Editors   124
  Frequencies   124
  Prices   124
  Scopes   124
  Telephone numbers   124
Health care
  Addresses   124
  Circulations   124
  Editors   124
  Frequencies   124
  Prices   124
  Scopes   124
  Telephone numbers   124
Medicine
  Addresses   124
  Circulations   124
  Editors   124
  Frequencies   124
  Prices   124
  Scopes   124
  Telephone numbers   124
Nursing
  Addresses   124
  Circulations   124
  Editors   124
  Frequencies   124
  Prices   124
  Scopes   124
  Telephone numbers   124
Pharmacology
  Addresses   124
  Circulations   124
  Editors   124
  Frequencies   124
  Prices   124
  Scopes   124
  Telephone numbers   124
Science
  Addresses   124
  Circulations   124
  Editors   124
  Frequencies   124
  Prices   124
  Scopes   124
  Telephone numbers   124
Veterinary medicine
  Addresses   124
  Circulations   124
  Editors   124
  Frequencies   124
  Prices   124

Scopes   124
  Telephone numbers   124
Biological sciences
  schools
  Addresses   341
  Chairpersons   341
  Expenses   341
  Faculty, number of   341
  Programs offered   341
  Students, number of   341
  Telephone numbers   341
  University community
  341
Biological scientists
  Addresses   23
  Birth dates   23
  Educational backgrounds
  23
  Marriage dates   23
  Memberships   23
  Professional experience
  23
  Specialties   23
Boards of nursing
  Addresses   296
  Telephone numbers   296
Burn centers   400
  Addresses   296
  Burn beds, number of
  296
  Directors   296
  Telephone numbers   296
Cancer protocols, experi-
  mental
  Dosage and administra-
  tion   87
  Entry criteria   87
  Investigators
    Addresses   87
    Telephone numbers   87
  Objectives   87
  Patient evaluation para-
  meters   87
  Patients allowed in pro-
  gram, number of   87
  Protocol outlines   87
Cancer research institutes
  Addresses   230
  Department heads   230
  Directors   230
  Financial data   230
  Patient statistical data
  230
  Personnel statistical
  data   230
  Professional educational

programs   230
Services   230
Telephone numbers   230
Telex numbers   230
Cancer treatment centers
Addresses   230
Department heads   230
Directors   230
Financial data   230
Patient statistical data
230
Personnel statistical
data   230
Professional educational
programs   230
Services   230
Telephone numbers   230
Telex numbers   230
Cancer treatment programs
Addresses   86
Descriptions   86
Hospital affiliations
86
Tabular data   86
Telephone numbers   86
Chemical distributors
Addresses   68
Telephone numbers   68
Telex numbers   68
Tollfree telephone num-
bers   68
TWX numbers   68
Congressional subcommit-
tees
Health care
Addresses   299
Birth dates   299
Birth places   299
Career biographies
299
Health staff aides
299
Photographs   299
Telephone numbers   299
Dental licensure
Certifying boards
Addresses   17
Contact persons   17
Dental schools
Academic calendars   10
Addresses   10, 36, 216,
341
Admission requirements
10, 36
Admission statistics   36
Chairpersons   341

Curricula   10, 36
Degrees awarded   10
Expenses   10, 36, 341
Facilities   36
Faculty, number of   341
Financial aid   10, 36
Programs offered   341
Selection criteria   10
Students, number of   341
Telephone numbers   341
University community
341
Federal information cen-
ters
Telephone numbers   129
Federal job information
centers
Addresses   129
Telephone numbers   129
Foundations   381
Activities   163
Addresses   163
Dates established   163
Donors   163
Financial data   163
Officials   163
Purposes   163
Telephone numbers   163
Trustees   163
Funeral service schools
Addresses   389
Programs offered   389
Telephone numbers   389
Governmental agencies
Abbreviations 151, 423
Acronyms   423
Activities   423
Addresses   151, 423
Founding dates   151
Functions   423
Health care
Activities   261
Addresses   261, 299
Directors   261
Officials   299
Telephone numbers
261, 299
History   423
Information sources   423
Members, numbers of   151
Officials   423
Organizational charts
423
Patient education   90
Staff, number of   151
Telephone numbers   151,

423
Health care services
  Administrators
    Addresses 440
    Biographical informa-
      tion 440
    Birth dates 440
    Educational back-
      grounds 440
    Places of birth 440
    Professional back-
      grounds 440
  Adoption 381
  Aged services 203, 381
  Alcoholism treatment
    programs 203
  Architects 381
  Awards 381
  Battered women services
    203
  Blind services 203
  Blood banks 381
  Clinics 203
  Community mental health
    centers 203
  Consulting firms 381
    Addresses 261
    Services 261
    Telephone numbers 261
  Contraception 381
  Coroners 381
  Counseling services 203
  Deaf services 203
  Diagnostic services 203
  Diseases
    Care programs 203
    Organizations 203
    Treatment programs
      203
  Emergency care 381
  Eye banks 203
  Family planning clinics
    203
  Forensic pathologists
    381
  Government health of-
    fices 381
  Grant programs
    Activities 261
    Addresses 261
  Handicapped aids 381
  Handicapped services
    381
  Handicapped special
    schools 381
  Health maintenance or-

ganizations 381
Home health agencies
  381
Hospices 203
Insurance companies 381
Laboratories 381
Legal services 381
Medical illustrators
  381
Medical writers 381
Medicare 381
Organ transplant regis-
  tries 381
Pain centers 203
Pediatric services
  Addresses 297
  Contact persons 297
  Telephone numbers 297
Public relations 381
Research centers 381
Runaway youth programs
  203
Sex counseling 381
Sex education 381
Smoking cessation pro-
  grams 203
Sudden infant death syn-
  drome centers 203
Treatment centers 203
Health systems agencies
  Executives
    Addresses 184
    Telephone numbers 184
Hospital administrators
  Addresses 123
  Awards 123
  Birth dates 123
  Birth places 123
  Educational backgrounds
    123
  Marital status 123
  Professional backgrounds
    123
  Telephone numbers 123
Hospitals
  Accreditation status
    184
  Addresses 184, 261,
    424
  Administrators 123,
    184, 424
  Admission statistics
    184
  Bassinets, number of
    184
  Beds, number of 184,

424
Births, number of   184
Census, average daily
  184
Facilities   184
Financial data   184
Nursing practice
  Employment possibili-
    ties   317
  Working conditions
    317
Occupancy, percentage of
  184
Personnel, number of
  184
Services   424
Specialized   381
Telephone numbers   184,
  261, 424
Hospitals, Canada
  Addresses   58
  Admission statistics   58
  Beds, number of   58
  Births, number of   58
  Department heads   58
  Financial data   58
  Ownership   58
  Telephone numbers   58
Hospitals, United Kingdom
  Addresses   268
  Beds, number of   268
  Department heads   268
  Telephone numbers   268
Information centers
  Addresses   129
  Directors   129
  Founding dates   129
  Holdings
    Statistical data   129
  Networks and consortia
    129
  Publications   129
  Services   129
  Special collections
    129
  Staff names   129
  Staff, number of   129
  Subjects   129
  Telephone numbers   129
Information services
  Addresses   150
  Clientele   150
  Directors   150
  Founding dates   150
  Functions   150
  Holdings   150

Input sources   150
Publications   150
Purposes   150
Services   150
Staff, number of   150
Telephone numbers   150
Information systems
  Addresses   150
  Clientele   150
  Directors   150
  Founding dates   150
  Functions   150
  Holdings   150
  Input sources   150
  Publications   150
  Purposes   150
  Services   150
  Staff, number of   150
  Telephone numbers   150
Job hunting
  Executive search firms
    Addresses   362
Journals
  Abstract services   420
  Addresses   420
  Bibliographic informa-
    tion   420
  Frequencies   420
  Indexing services   420
  ISSN's   420
  Ordering information
    420
  Telephone numbers   420
Journals, medical
  Addresses   261, 265
  Frequencies   261
Journals, medical, United
  Kingdom
  Addresses   268
Laboratories
  Addresses   424
  Services   424
  Telephone numbers   424
Libraries for the blind
  Addresses   129, 261
  Directors   129
  Telephone numbers   129,
    261
Libraries, medical
  Addresses   125, 261
  Data base access   125
  Directors   125, 261
  Holdings
    Statistical data   125,
      261
  Personnel

Statistical data   125
Sponsoring organizations
   125
Telephone numbers   261
Libraries, research
   Addresses   129
   Directors   129
   Founding dates   129
   Holdings   129
   Networks and consortia
      129
   Publications   129
   Services   129
   Special collections   129
   Staff names   129
   Staff, numbers of   129
   Telephone numbers   129
Libraries, special
   Addresses   129
   Directors   129
   Founding dates   129
   Holdings   129
   Networks and consortia
      129
   Publications   129
   Services   129
   Special collections   129
   Staff names   129
   Staff, number of   129
   Telephone numbers   129
Libraries, world
   Addresses   445
   Directors   445
   Holdings   445
Library networks
   Addresses   129
   Directors   129
   Telephone numbers   129
Manufacturers, chemicals
   Addresses   68
   Telephone numbers   68
   Telex numbers   68
   Tollfree telephone num-
      bers   68
   TWX numbers   68
Manufacturers, drugs
   Addresses   18, 19, 136,
      348, 349, 429
   Calendars, merchandising
      136
   Catalogs   19, 136
   Contact persons   348,
      349
   Identification   19
   National drug code num-
      bers   19

Packaging   19
Prices   19
Return policies   136
Telephone numbers   136,
   348, 349
Manufacturers, drugs, Eu-
ropean
   Addresses   257
Manufacturers, drugs,
veterinary medicine
   Addresses   434
Manufacturers, equipment,
medical
   Addresses   263
   Distributors   263
   Employees, number of
      263
   Financial data   263
   Officials   263
   Sales statistics   263
   Telephone numbers   263
Manufacturers, laboratory
equipment
   Addresses   183
   Telephone numbers   183
Manufacturers, laboratory
instruments
   Addresses   183
   Telephone numbers   183
Manufacturers, medical
products
   Addresses   263
   Distributors   263
   Employees, number of
      263
   Financial data   263
   Officials   263
   Sales statistics   263
   Telephone numbers   263
Medic alert   203
Medical examination
boards, state
   Addresses   424
   Telephone numbers   424
Medical licensing boards,
state
   Addresses   424
   Telephone numbers   424
Medical schools
   Academic calendars   1,
      275
   Addresses   1, 2, 36,
      261, 275, 341, 424
   Admission requirements
      36, 275
   Admission statistics   36

UF-Used For, BT-Broader Term, NT-Narrower Term, RT-Related Term

Chairpersons 341
Clinical facilities 2
Curricula 1, 36, 275
Deans 261
Enrollment data 2
Expenses 36, 275, 341
Facilities 36
Faculty, number of 341
Financial aid 36, 275
Founding dates 2
Officials 2, 275
Programs offered 341
Selection factors 275
Statistical data 275
Students, number of 341
Telephone numbers 1, 2,
  261, 275, 341
University community
  341
Medical schools, foreign
Addresses 36, 261, 442
Admission requirements
  36
Admission statistics
  442
Enrollment, number of
  442
Faculty, number of 442
Founding dates 442
Graduates, number of
  442
Language of instruction
  442
Students, number of 442
Medical schools, United
Kingdom
Addresses 268
Administrators 268
Department heads 268
Telephone numbers 268
Medical specialists
Addresses 126
Birth dates 126
Birth places 126
Educational backgrounds
  126
Professional backgrounds
  126
Professional certifica-
  tions 126
Telephone numbers 126
Meetings, future
Medicine
  Attendees, estimated
    number of 444
  Contact persons 444

Dates 444
Exhibit information
  444
Languages 444
Locations 444
Paper submission dead-
  lines 444
Proceedings, sources
  of 444
Sponsors 444
Subject content 444
Translation facilities
  444
Mental health services
Pediatrics
  Addresses 297
  Contact persons 297
  Telephone numbers 297
Migrant health centers
  203
Multihospital systems
Addresses 184
Executives 184
Telephone numbers 184
Museums, world
Addresses 445
Directors 445
Holdings 445
Nursing
Certification 303
Education 303
Federal health offices
  303
Licensure 303
State health offices
  303
Nursing homes
Addresses 424
Administrators 424
Beds, number of 424
Services 424
Nursing schools
Addresses 341
Chairpersons 341
Directories 303
Expenses 341
Faculty, number of 341
Information sources 303
Programs offered 341
Ratings 176
Statistical data 303
Students, number of 341
Telephone numbers 341
University community
  341
Organizations

Activities 446
Addresses 446
Conferences 446
Dates founded 446
Financial data 446
Languages 446
Members, number of 446
Patient education 90
Publications 446
Staff, number of 446
Organizations, dental
Activities 151
Addresses 17, 151
Contact persons 17
Founding dates 151
Members, number of 151
Staff, number of 151
Telephone numbers 151
Organizations, health care
381
Acronyms 147
Activities 147, 198
Addresses 58, 147, 184,
198, 261
Awards 198
Descriptions 198, 261
Directors 261
Founding dates 147, 198
Journals 261
Meetings 147, 198
Members, number of 147,
261
Membership fees 198
Membership statistics
198
Officials 147
Publications 147, 198
Telephone numbers 58,
147, 184, 198, 261
Organizations, medical
Acronyms 147
Activities 147, 151
Addresses 147, 151, 261
Descriptions 261
Directors 261
Founding dates 147,
151
Journals 261
Meeting dates 147
Meeting locations 147
Members, number of 147,
151, 261
Officials 147
Publications 147
Staff, number of 151
Telephone numbers 147,

151, 261
Organizations, nursing
303
Activities 151, 157
Addresses 151, 157,
296
Founding dates 151
Members, number of 151
Staff, number of 151
Telephone numbers 151
Organizations, pharmaco-
logical
Activities 151
Addresses 136, 151
Contact persons 136
Founding dates 151
Members, number of 151
Staff, number of 151
Telephone numbers 136,
151
Organizations, scientific
Acronyms 147
Activities 147
Addresses 147
Founding dates 147
Meeting dates 147
Meeting locations 147
Members, number of 147
Officials 147
Publications 147
Telephone numbers 147
Patent depository librar-
ies
Addresses 129
Telephone numbers 129
Patient education
Audiovisual producers
Addresses 90
Governmental agencies
Addresses 90
Insurance companies
Addresses 90
Organizations
Addresses 90
Publishers
Addresses 90
Voluntary health organi-
zations
Addresses 90
Pediatrics
Services
Addresses 297
Contact persons 297
Telephone numbers 297
Pharmacists
Activities, research

343
  Addresses 343
  Birth dates 343
  Career backgrounds 343
  Educational backgrounds
    343
  Professional memberships
    343
  Publications 343
  Telephone numbers 343
Pharmacy schools
  Addresses 341
  Chairpersons 341
  Expenses 341
  Faculty, number of 341
  Programs offered 341
  Students, number of 341
  Telephone numbers 341
  University community
    341
Physical scientists
  Addresses 23
  Birth dates 23
  Educational backgrounds
    23
  Marriage dates 23
  Memberships 23
  Professional experience
    23
  Specialties 23
Physicians
  Addresses 22, 424
  American specialty board
    certification 22, 424
  Birth dates 424
  Certification 22, 424
  Educational backgrounds
    22, 424
  Practice types 22
  Professional memberships
    424
  Specialties 22, 126,
    424
  Year of licensure 22
Physicians, United Kingdom
  Addresses 268, 274
  Dates of registration
    274
  Professional degrees
    268
  Professional member-
    ships 268
  Registration numbers
    274
  Telephone numbers 268
Physicians, women

  Addresses 130
  Educational backgrounds
    130
  Professional backgrounds
    130
  Specialties 126, 130
Poison control centers
  400
  Addresses 225, 261,
    296, 348, 349
  Telephone numbers 225,
    261, 296, 348, 349
Public health schools
  Addresses 46, 341
  Chairpersons 341
  Deans 46
  Expenses 341
  Faculty, number of 341
  Programs offered 341
  Students, number of 341
  Telephone numbers 341
  University community
    341
Public health scientists
  Addresses 23
  Birth dates 23
  Educational backgrounds
    23
  Marriage dates 23
  Memberships 23
  Professional experience
    23
  Specialties 23
Publishers 381
  Books
    Addresses 265
    Telephone numbers 265
  Journals
    Addresses 265, 420
    Telephone numbers 420
Research centers
  Addresses 375
  Dates founded 375
  Directors 375
  Facilities 375
  Financial data 375
  Library facilities 375
  Parent institutions 375
  Publications 375
  Research activities 375
  Staff, number of 375
  Support sources 375
  Telephone numbers 375
Research institutes, for-
  eign
  Addresses 445

Officials   445
Publications   445
Telephone numbers   445
Research programs
   Allied health sciences
      Addresses   376
      Cable addresses   376
      Officials   376
      Research activities
         376
      Staff, number of   376
      Telephone numbers   376
      Telex numbers   376
      TWX numbers   376
   Biomedical sciences
      Addresses   376
      Cable addresses   376
      Officials   376
      Research activities
         376
      Staff, number of   376
      Telephone numbers   376
      Telex numbers   376
      TWX numbers   376
   Dentistry
      Addresses   376
      Cable addresses   376
      Officials   376
      Research activities
         376
      Staff, number of   376
      Telephone numbers   376
      Telex numbers   376
      TWX numbers   376
   Medical sciences
      Addresses   376
      Cable addresses   376
      Officials   376
      Research activities
         376
      Staff, number of   376
      Telephone numbers   376
      Telex numbers   376
      TWX numbers   376
   Pharmacology
      Addresses   376
      Cable addresses   376
      Officials   376
      Research activities
         376
      Staff, number of   376
      Telephone numbers   376
      Telex numbers   376
      TWX numbers   376
   Veterinary medicine
      Addresses   376

      Cable addresses   376
      Officials   376
      Research activities
         376
      Staff, number of   376
      Telephone numbers   376
      Telex numbers   376
      TWX numbers   376
Residency programs, ac-
   credited
   Addresses   128
   Admissions, annual   128
   Affiliations, medical
      schools   128
   Autopsies, percentage of
      128
   Beds, number of   128
   Census, average daily
      128
   Medical education direc-
      tors   128
   Medical staff, number in
      128
   Program directors   128
Runaway youth centers
   Addresses   297
   Contact persons   297
   Telephone numbers   297
Senators and representa-
   tives
   Addresses   299
   Aides, health issues
      299
   Appointment secretaries
      299
   District offices
      Addresses   299
      Contact persons   299
      Telephone numbers   299
   Health committee member-
      ship   299
   Health subcommittee mem-
      bership   299
   Telephone numbers   299
Tel-Med   203
Treatment facilities
   Pediatrics
      Addresses   297
      Contact persons   297
      Telephone numbers   297
Universities, world
   Addresses   445
   Dates founded   445
   Faculty members   445
   Faculty, number of   445

UF–Used For, BT–Broader Term, NT–Narrower Term, RT–Related Term

Students, number of 445
Telephone numbers 445
Veterinary medicine
schools
    Addresses 341
    Chairpersons 341
    Expenses 341
    Faculty, number of 341
    Programs offered 341
    Students, number of 341
    Telephone numbers 341
    University community
    341

DIRECTORS

RT Administrators
RT Chairpersons
RT Contact persons
RT Deans
RT Department heads
RT Officials
 Archives 129
 Burn centers 296
 Cancer research institutes
 230
 Cancer treatment centers
 230
 Governmental agencies
   Health care 261
 Information centers 129
 Information services 150
 Information systems 150
 Libraries for the blind
 129
 Libraries, medical 125,
 261
 Libraries, research 129
 Libraries, special 129
 Libraries, world 445
 Library networks 129
 Museums, world 445
 Organizations, health
 care 198, 261
 Organizations, medical
 261
 Research centers 375

DISABILITY, PHYSICAL

RT Handicapped services
 Diagnosis 237
 Neurophysiology
   Motor functions 237
 Occupational health 237
 Physical therapy 237

Plastic surgery 237
Psychological aspects 237
Rehabilitation 237

DISEASES

UF Abnormalities
UF Disorders
NT Cancer
NT Communicable diseases
NT Coronary artery dis-
    eases
NT Diabetes
NT Syndromes
RT Acid-base disturbances
RT Body fluid disturbances
RT Electrolyte distur-
    bances
RT Mental illness
 Abdomen
   Diagnosis 4
   Signs and symptoms 4
   Treatment, surgical 4
 Adrenals
   Diagnosis 57
   Signs and symptoms 57
   Treatment 57
 Aged
   Diagnosis 72
   Treatment 72
 Alimentary tract
   Treatment, surgical 393
 Allergy
   Diagnosis 12
   Drugs (treatment modal-
   ity)
     Adverse effects 12
     Dosage and administra-
     tion 12
     Pharmacokinetics 12
     Pharmacology 12
     Toxicology 12
   Signs and symptoms 12
 Ambulatory medicine
   Diagnosis 358
   Epidemiology 358
   Etiology 358
   Pathogenesis 358
   Physical examination
   358
   Prognosis 358
   Signs and symptoms 358
   Treatment 358
 Animal hosts
   Handbooks
     Laboratory animal sci-

ences 97
Animals
  Diagnosis 131
  Encyclopedias 146
  Treatment 131
Anus
  Signs and symptoms 394
  Treatment, surgical
  393, 394
Atlases 70, 181
Bibliographies
  History 42
  Mendelian inheritance
  284
Bile ducts
  Diagnosis 132, 133
  Pathology 133
  Signs and symptoms 132,
  133
  Treatment 132, 133
Biliary ducts, extrahepatic
  Treatment, surgical 393
Biochemistry 415
  Pathophysiology 403
Blood vessels
  Anesthesia 205
  Diagnosis 205
  Pathophysiology 205
  Signs and symptoms 205
  Treatment 205
Body fluid disturbances
  Biochemistry 74
  Diagnosis 74
  Pathophysiology 74
  Physiology 74
  Treatment 74
Cardiovascular system
  Diagnosis 417
  Pathophysiology 417
  Treatment, surgical
    Anatomy 417
    Anesthesia 417
    Postoperative care
    417
    Preoperative care 417
    Techniques 417
Charges
  Quality assurance standards
    Hospitals 332
Child psychiatry
  Diagnosis 89
  Epidemiology 89
  Etiology 89
  Signs and symptoms 89

Treatment 89
Classification systems
229, 398
Colon
  Signs and symptoms 394
  Treatment, surgical
  393, 394
Dentistry
  Diagnosis
    Instruments 345
    Techniques 345
  Drugs (treatment modality)
    Actions and uses 5
    Adverse effects 5
    Chemical descriptions
    5
    Distributors 5
    Trade names 5
    Warnings 5
  Prevention 5
Dentistry, operative
  Cavity preparation 320
  Diagnosis 320
  Pulp protection 320
  Restorations 320
  Treatment planning 320
Dermatology
  Atlases 116, 256
  Classification systems
  116, 256
  Descriptions 256
  Diagnosis 26, 116, 256
  Diagnosis, laboratory
  26, 256
  Differential diagnosis
  26, 256
  Encyclopedias, loose-
  leaf 81
  Epidemiology 26, 116
  Etiology 26, 256
  Histopathology 26
  Natural histories 256
  Pathogenesis 26, 116
  Pathology 116
  Pathophysiology 26
  Prevention 116
  Prognosis 116
  Signs and symptoms 26,
  116
  Treatment 26, 116, 256
Dictionaries
  Etiology 217
  Inheritance 217
  Original articles
    Bibliographies 217

UF—Used For, BT—Broader Term, NT—Narrower Term, RT—Related Term

Pathology   217
Signs and symptoms   50,
  217
Synonyms   217
Treatment   50
Drugs of choice   139
Duodenum
  Treatment, surgical   393
Electrolyte disturbances
  Biochemistry   74
  Diagnosis   74, 372, 392
  Metabolism   74
  Pathogenesis   372
  Pathophysiology   74, 392
  Physiology   74, 392
  Signs and symptoms   372,
    392
  Treatment   74, 372, 392
Emergency care
  Assessment, prehospital
    143
  Classification systems
    143
  Diagnosis   142, 143
  Diagnosis, radiologic
    367
  Differential diagnosis
    142
  Etiology   142, 143
  History and physical ex-
    amination   143
  Indications for admis-
    sion   142
  Pathology   142
  Pathophysiology   142,
    143
  Pediatrics
    Differential diagnosis
      412
    Drugs (treatment mo-
      dality)   412
    Pathophysiology   412
    Signs and symptoms
      412
    Treatment   412
  Signs and symptoms   143
  Stabilization, emergency
    room   143
  Treatment   142, 143
Encyclopedias
  Diagnosis   196
  Etiology   196
  Pathophysiology   196
  Signs and symptoms   196
  Treatment   196
Encyclopedias, loose-leaf

Classification   81
Complications   81
Definitions   81
Diagnosis   81
Etiology   81
History   81
Incidence   81
Pathology   81
Pathophysiology   81
Signs and symptoms   81
Treatment   81
Endocrine system
  Diagnosis   76, 153, 405
  Etiology   153
  Gynecology   76
  Pathology   405
  Physiology   76
  Signs and symptoms   153,
    405
  Treatment   76, 153, 405
Esophagus
  Treatment, surgical   393
Family medicine
  Diagnosis   406
  Pathology   406
  Signs and symptoms   406
  Treatment   406
Gallbladder
  Diagnosis   132, 133
  Pathology   133
  Signs and symptoms   132,
    133
  Treatment   132, 133
  Treatment, surgical   393
Gastrointestinal system
  Complications   169
  Diagnosis   75, 168, 169
    Pediatrics   335
  Epidemiology   169
  Etiology   75, 169
  Incidence   75
  Pathogenesis   75
    Pediatrics   335
  Pathology   75, 169
  Pathophysiology   75,
    168, 169
  Signs and symptoms   75,
    168, 169
    Pediatrics   335
  Treatment   75, 168, 169
    Pediatrics   335
Genetics
  Diagnosis   270, 287
  Diagnosis, laboratory
    287
  Differential diagnosis

270
Etiology   270
Fetus
  Diagnosis   270
Incidence   270
Metabolism   287
Pathogenesis   287
Pathophysiology   287
Signs and symptoms   270,
  287
Treatment   270, 287
Genitourinary system
  Complications   172
  Diagnosis   172
  Etiology   172
  Pathogenesis   172
  Prognosis   172
  Signs and symptoms   172
  Treatment   172
Genitourinary system,
  female
  Diagnosis   185
  Signs and symptoms   185
  Treatment   185
Gynecology
  Adolescence   186
  Classification systems
    191
  Complications   191
  Diagnosis   76, 106, 311,
    318
  Differential diagnosis
    191
  Endocrine system   76,
    310
  Pathology   191, 310, 311
  Physiology   76
  Prognosis   191
  Signs and symptoms   106,
    191, 310, 311, 318
    Pediatrics   186
  Treatment   76, 106, 191,
    311, 318
    Pediatrics   186
  Treatment, surgical
    Complications   401
    Hyperalimentation   401
    Postoperative care
      401
    Preoperative care   401
    Techniques   401
  Urology   185
Handbooks
  Complications   105
  Diagnosis   104, 105,
    253, 286

Differential diagnosis
  104, 105
Epidemiology   104
Etiology   104, 286
Prevention   286
Prognosis   105, 286
Signs and symptoms   104,
  105, 111, 253, 286
Treatment   105, 111,
  253, 286
Heart
  Anesthesia   205, 206
  Complications   206
  Diagnosis   173, 205, 206
  Echocardiography   140
  Pathophysiology   205,
    206
  Pregnancy   206
  Psychiatric aspects   206
  Signs and symptoms   205,
    206
  Treatment   173, 205, 206
  Treatment, surgical   173
Hematology
  Diagnosis   77, 207
  Diagnosis, laboratory
    207
    Atlases   240
    Equipment   240
    Normal ranges   240
    Reagents   240
    Techniques   240
  Differential diagnosis
    77
  Etiology   77, 207
  Pathogenesis   77, 207,
    240
  Pediatrics   208
  Prognosis   207
  Signs and symptoms   77,
    207, 240
  Treatment   77, 207
Histopathology
  Veterinary medicine
    Cats   416
    Dogs   416
History
  Bibliographies, annota-
    ted
    Medicine   264
  Indexes, literature   42
  Original descriptions
    71
    Physician biographies
      (authors)   71
Immunology   73, 415

Complications 37
Diagnosis, immunologic
  37
Differential diagnosis
  37
Prevention 37
Prognosis 37
Signs and symptoms 37
Treatment 37
Indications for admission
  Quality assurance stan-
    dards
    Hospitals 332
Indications for diagnostic
tests
  Quality assurance stan-
    dards
    Hospitals 332
Indications for discharge
  Quality assurance stan-
    dards
    Hospitals 332
Indications for treatment
  Quality assurance stan-
    dards
    Hospitals 332
Kidneys
  Diagnosis 236, 392
  Epidemiology 236
  Etiology 236
  Pathogenesis 236
  Pathophysiology 236,
    392
  Physiology 392
  Signs and symptoms 236,
    392
  Treatment 236, 392
Length of stay
  Quality assurance stan-
    dards
    Hospitals 332
Liver
  Diagnosis 132, 133
  Epidemiology 132
  Etiology 132, 133
  Pathogenesis 372
  Pathology 132, 133
  Prognosis 133
  Signs and symptoms 132,
    133
  Treatment 132, 133, 372
  Treatment, surgical 393
Medical firsts
  Bibliographies 152
Metabolism 217, 288
  Diagnosis, radiologic

  368
Differential diagnosis
  368
Modes of inheritance
  368
Oral manifestations 410
Original articles
  Bibliographies 368
Signs and symptoms 368
Morphology 329
Mouth
  Examination techniques
    324
  Histology 410
  Prognosis 410
  Signs and symptoms 324,
    410
  Treatment 324, 410
Nervous system
  Diagnosis 92, 306, 408
  Differential diagnosis
    92
  Encyclopedias, loose-
    leaf 82
  Etiology 306, 408
  Incidence 408
  Nursing practice
    Classification sys-
      tems 63
    Diagnosis 63
    History and physical
      examination 63
    Prognosis 63
  Pathogenesis 306
  Pathology 408
  Prognosis 306
  Signs and symptoms 359,
    408
  Treatment 306, 408
  Treatment, surgical 306
Neuro-ophthalmology
  Etiology 171
  Signs and symptoms 171
Newborns
  Diagnosis 382
  Etiology 382
  Incidence 382
  Pathophysiology 305
  Prognosis 382
  Signs and symptoms 382
  Treatment 305, 382
Nursing practice
  Diagnosis 242
  Drugs (treatment modal-
    ity)
    Actions and uses 160

Adverse effects 160
Chemical properties
  160
Dosage and adminis-
  tration 160
Interactions 160
Pharmacokinetics 160
Physical properties
  160
Preparations 160
Toxicology
  Treatment 160
Warnings 160
Etiology 242
Incubation periods 144
Nervous system 63
Ophthalmology 316
Otolaryngology 316
Patient advice 242
Patient care standards
  333
Signs and symptoms 242,
  333
Treatment 242
Obstetrics
Endocrine system 310
Pathology 310
Signs and symptoms 310
Treatment 441
Ocular manifestations 323
Ophthalmology
Classification systems
  171
Diagnosis 322, 323
  Pediatrics 336
Etiology 171
Pathology 171
Prognosis 171
Signs and symptoms 171,
  323
  Nursing practice 316
  Pediatrics 336
Treatment 171, 323
  Pediatrics 336
Treatment, surgical 322
Original articles
Bibliographies 152
Orthopedics
Anatomy 327
Diagnosis 326
  Pediatrics 337
Diagnosis, radiologic
  327
Dictionaries 254
Etiology 326, 327
Pathogenesis 327

Pathology 326
  Pediatrics 337
Prognosis 327
Signs and symptoms 326
  Pediatrics 337
Treatment 326, 327
  Pediatrics 337
Treatment, surgical 56
Otolaryngology
Diagnosis 328, 411
Etiology 328
Pathology 328
Signs and symptoms 328
  Nursing practice 316
Treatment 328, 411
Pancreas
Treatment, surgical 393
Parasitology
Diagnosis 83, 168
Pathogenesis 83
Pathology 83
Prevention 83
Prognosis 83
Signs and symptoms 83
Treatment 83, 168
Patient education
Activity restrictions
  227
Descriptions 227
Diet therapy 227
Drugs, nonprescription
  190
Handbooks
  Family practice 281
Medication instructions
  227
Medication precautions
  227
Warning signs of compl-
  ications 227
Pediatrics
Complications 339
Diagnosis 108, 192,
  304, 339, 439
  Nursing practice 88
Diagnosis, laboratory
  Indications 232
  Interferences, drug
    232
  Interpretations 232
Diagnosis, radiologic
  338
Differential diagnosis
  108, 192
Emergency care 412
Epidemiology 339

UF-Used For, BT-Broader Term, NT-Narrower Term, RT-Related Term

Etiology   304, 339
Gastrointestinal system
 335
Hematology   208
Ocular manifestations
 336
Ophthalmology   336
Orthopedics   337
Pathology   304, 339
Prevention   304, 339
Prognosis   108, 192,
 304, 339
Signs and symptoms   108,
 192, 304, 339
 Nursing practice   88
Techniques   195, 412
Treatment   108, 109,
 192, 304, 339
 Nursing practice   88
Treatment, surgical   397
Pregnancy   266
Diagnosis
 Nursing practice   258
Psychiatric manifestations
 291
Psychiatry
Classification systems
 89
Diagnosis   89
Drugs (treatment modal-
 ity)   89
Epidemiology   89
Etiology   89
Residential care   89
Signs and symptoms   89
Treatment   89
Rectum
Signs and symptoms   394
Treatment, surgical
 393, 394
Respiratory system
Diagnosis   173, 365,
 366, 413
 Techniques   365
Diagnosis, radiologic
 117
Differential diagnosis
 Decision trees   117
Etiology   117, 365, 413
Pathogenesis   117, 413
Pathology   117, 365
Physiology   365, 413
Prognosis   365
Signs and symptoms   117,
 365, 366
Treatment   173, 365,

366, 413
Treatment, surgical
 173
Rheumatology
Diagnosis   31, 84, 414
Diagnosis, radiologic
 31
Differential diagnosis
 31, 84
Drugs (treatment modal-
 ity)   84
 Adverse effects   31,
  414
 Dosage and administra-
  tion   31, 414
 Indications   31, 414
 Pharmacokinetics   31,
  414
 Toxicology   31, 414
Epidemiology   31
Etiology   31, 414
Examination   84
Immunopathology   31
Occupational therapy   84
Pathogenesis   31
Pathology   31, 414
Pathophysiology   31
Physical therapy   84
Rehabilitation   414
Signs and symptoms   31,
 84, 414
Treatment   31, 84, 414
Sexuality   89
Spleen
Treatment, surgical   393
Stomach
Treatment, surgical   393
Thorax
Diagnosis   173, 417
Pathophysiology   417
Treatment   173
Treatment, surgical   173
 Anatomy   417
 Anesthesia   417
 Postoperative care
  417
 Preoperative care   417
 Techniques   417
Urology
Diagnosis   57
Etiology   57
Gynecology   185
Obstetrics   185
Signs and symptoms   57,
 112
Treatment   57, 112

Treatment, surgical   57
Veterinary medicine
  Autopsies
    Cattle 432
    Horses 432
    Pigs 432
    Sheep 432
  Control
    Cattle 432
    Horses 432
    Pigs 432
    Sheep 432
  Diagnosis
    Cats 416
    Cattle 432
    Dogs 416
    Horses 432
    Pigs 432
    Sheep 432
    Amall animals 113
  Drugs (treatment modal-
  ity)
    Contraindications 435
    Indications 435
    Physical description
    435
    Toxicology 435
    Uses 435
    Warnings 435
  Etiology
    Cats 416
    Cattle 432
    Dogs 416
    Horses 432
    Pigs 432
    Sheep 432
    Small animals 113
  Pathogenesis
    Cattle 432
    Horses 432
    Pigs 432
    Sheep 432
  Pathology 433
    Cattle 432
    Horses 432
    Pigs 432
    Sheep 432
  Pathophysiology
    Small animals 113
  Prognosis
    Small animals 113
  Signs and symptoms 51
    Cats 416
    Cattle 432
    Dogs 416
    Horses 432

    Pigs 432
    Sheep 432
    Small animals 113
  Treatment
    Cats 416
    Cattle 432
    Dogs 416
    Horses 432
    Pigs 432
    Sheep 432
    Small animals 113

DISLOCATIONS

  RT Orthopedics
    Atlases 115
    Classification systems
    165
    Complications 165
    Diagnosis 115, 165
    Dictionaries 254
    Historical backgrounds
    165
    Mechanism of injury 115
      Pediatrics 337
    Pathological anatomy 165
      Pediatrics 337
    Treatment 115, 165
      Pediatrics 337
    Treatment, surgical 56

DISORDERS

  See Diseases

DIVORCES

  RT Family medicine
  RT Marriage
    Statistical data 436,
    437

DIZZINESS

  Differential diagnosis
  244

DOGS

  BT Animals
  Diseases
    Diagnosis 416
    Etiology 416
    Histopathology 416
    Signs and symptoms 416
    Treatment 416

Normal laboratory values
113
Physiology 416

DOSAGE AND ADMINISTRATION

UF Administration (drugs)
UF Routes of administra-
    tion (drugs)
RT Packaging
Antibiotic drugs 105
Antimicrobial drugs 105
Cancer protocols, experi-
  mental 87
Drugs 15, 18, 20, 136,
  138, 158, 175, 188, 298,
  350, 371, 426, 428
  Nursing practice 62,
    137, 144, 160, 295,
    312, 313
  Pediatrics 195, 304,
    336, 412
  Veterinary medicine 434
Drugs, European 257
Drugs, injectable 194
Drugs, new 138, 344, 422
Drugs, nonprescription
  349
Drugs, prescription 348
Drugs (treatment modality)
  30
  Allergy 12
  Cancer 79
  Communicable diseases
    355
  Emergency care 290, 412
  Ophthalmology 336
  Rheumatology 31, 414
Drugs, United Kingdom 55
English-Spanish glossaries
  280
Immunizations 253
Patient education 21, 280

DRUG ABUSE

NT Alcohol abuse
RT Drugs
Adolescence
  Treatment 109
Family practice 281
Medicolegal investiga-
  tions 292
Pregnancy 266
Psychiatry 291
  Diagnosis 89

Signs and symptoms 89
Treatment 89
Signs and symptoms
  Encyclopedias, loose-
    leaf
    Nervous system 82
Treatment
  Encyclopedias, loose-
    leaf
    Nervous system 82
Withdrawal
  Adverse effects 289

DRUG INTERACTIONS

UF Interactions
BT Adverse effects
RT Cross-sensitivity
RT Food-drug interactions
Drugs 15, 20, 135, 136,
  156, 158, 175, 188, 289,
  371, 427, 428
  Nursing practice 137,
    160, 312, 313
  Prevention 156
Drugs, nonprescription
  349
Food-drug interactions
  Nursing practice 137

DRUG INTERFERENCES

See Interferences

DRUG MANUFACTURERS

See Manufacturers, drugs

DRUG RESPONSE VARIATION

Drugs 15

DRUG STORE MERCHANDISE

RT Commercial products,
    chemicals
RT Cosmetics
RT Household products
Catalogs
  Biologicals
    Prices (retail &
      wholesale) 136
  Botanicals
    Prices (retail &
      wholesale) 136
  Cosmetics

Prices (retail &
wholesale) 136
Fountain products
Prices (retail &
wholesale) 136
Perfumes
Prices (retail &
wholesale) 136
Pharmaceuticals
Prices (retail &
wholesale) 136
Stationery
Prices (retail &
wholesale) 136

DRUGS

BT   Chemicals
NT   Antibiotic drugs
NT   Antimicrobial drugs
NT   Drugs, British
NT   Drugs, European
NT   Drugs, immunosuppres-
sive
NT   Drugs, injectable
NT   Drugs, new
NT   Drugs, nonprescription
NT   Drugs of choice
NT   Drugs, prescription
NT   Ear drops
NT   Eye drops
NT   Eye ointments
NT   Investigational drugs
NT   Nose drops
NT   Rectal suppositories
RT   Drug abuse
RT   Drugs (treatment modal-
ity)
RT   Manufacturers, drugs
RT   Manufacturers, drugs,
veterinary medicine
RT   Pharmaceutical ingredi-
ents
RT   Pharmaceutical practice
RT   Pharmacology
Actions and uses 15, 18,
20, 136, 138, 158, 175,
285, 298, 313, 371, 428,
429
Adverse effects 15, 20,
50, 136, 138, 156, 158,
175, 289, 371, 428
Bibliographies 289
Pediatrics 195
Withdrawal effects 289
AMA evaluations 15

Assays 426
Brand names 18, 20, 138,
158, 428, 429
Breast feeding 20, 296,
428
Recommendations 232
Warnings 232
Carcinogenicity 20
CAS registry numbers 285,
429
Catalogs
Adverse effects 136
Atlases 136
Descriptions 136
Drug interactions
136
Indications 136
Packaging 136
Changed products
Discontinued drug rein-
troduced 344
New dosage forms 344
New manufacturers 344
New packaging 344
Chemical characteristics
426
Chemical names 18, 429
Synonyms 342
Chemistry 20, 175
Classification systems
298
Composition 18, 285
Cost (wholesale) 158
Cross-sensitivity 428
Descriptions 138, 344
Distributors 298
Dosage and administration
15, 18, 20, 136, 138,
158, 175, 298, 313, 371,
426, 428
English-Spanish glossa-
ries 280
Handbooks
Pediatrics 195
Drug interactions 15, 20,
158, 175, 289, 371, 428
Clinical data 156
Dosage and administra-
tion 156
Pharmacology 156
Prevention 156
Related drugs 156
Drug response variation
15
Drugs of choice 15
Generic names 18, 21,

156, 158, 429
Handbooks
  Pediatrics   195
Handbooks
  Adverse effects   188,
    350
  Biopharmaceuticals   188
  Dosage and administra-
    tion   188, 350
  Monitoring parameters
    188
  Patient education   188
  Pharmacokinetics   188
  Pharmacology   188
History   175
Identification tests   426
Indications   138, 158, 428
  Handbooks
    Pediatrics   195
Interferences   20, 231,
  289, 428
  Nursing practice   239
  Pediatrics   232
Molecular formulas   285,
  371, 426, 429
Molecular weights   285,
  429
Name changes   18
National drug codes   298
Natural ingredients
  Chemical composition
    149
  Commercially available
    forms   149
  Pharmacology   149
  Physical descriptions
    149
  Plant sources   149
  Preparation methods   149
  Synonyms   149
New products
  Adverse effects   344
  Descriptions   344
  Dosage and administra-
    tion   344
  Indications   344
  Pharmacology   344
  Related products   344
  Warnings   344
Nursing practice
  Actions and uses   137,
    144, 160, 312, 313
  Adverse effects   137,
    160, 312, 313
    Classification systems
      229

Brand names
  Actions and uses   313
  Dosage and administra-
    tion   313
  Formulas   313
  Legal status   313
  Manufacturers, drugs
    313
Breast feeding   137
Classification systems
  312
Dispensing instructions
  313
Dosage and administra-
  tion   137, 144, 160,
  312, 313
Drug interactions   137,
  312, 313
Food-drug interactions
  137
Generic names   160
Interferences   137, 312,
  313
Legal status   313
Overdosage
  Treatment   313
Patient education   137,
  313
Pharmacokinetics 137,
  160, 175
Pharmacology   313
Pregnancy   137
Preparations   144, 160
Pronunciations   137
Storage requirements
  312, 313
Synonyms   160
Trade names   137, 160
Uses, emergency   144
Overdosage   158
Patient education
  Actions and uses   280,
    427
  Adverse effects   21,
    280, 427
  Brand names   427
  Breast feeding   427
  Dosage and administra-
    tion   21, 280
  Drug interactions   427
  Generic names   21
  Nursing practice   137,
    313
  Pregnancy   427
  Pronunciations   427
  Storage recommendations

280
Trade names 21
Pediatrics 195
Pharmacokinetics 15, 20,
138, 158, 175, 428
Pharmacological names
Synonyms 342
Pharmacology 20, 286
Physical characteristics
426
Physical descriptions 371
Physical properties 138
Poisoning
Diagnosis 193, 351
Prevention 193
Prognosis 193
Signs and symptoms 193,
351
Treatment 138, 193, 351
Pregnancy 20, 296, 428
Prices 19, 136
Product identification
numbers 158
Pronunciations 280, 429
Reference standards 426
Solubility 371, 426
Stability 20
Storage 426
Strengths 18, 298
Structural formulas 15,
20, 175, 285, 371, 426,
429
Synonyms 138, 285, 342
Teratogenic agents
Abstracts, literature
64
Indexes, literature 64
Toxicology 20, 138, 175,
285
Trade names 15, 156, 298
Handbooks
Pediatrics 195
Synonyms 342
Trademarks 285
Veterinary medicine
Actions and uses 51,
434
Adverse effects 434
Composition 434
Dosage and administra-
tion 434
Forms of distribution
434
Identification
Color illustrations
434

Indications 434

DRUGS, BRITISH

BT   Drugs
BT   Chemicals, European
RT   Drugs, European
Actions and uses 55
Chemical properties 55
Dosage and administration
55
Identification techniques
55
Molecular formulas 55
Physical descriptions 55
Physical properties   55
Preparations 55
Solubility 55
Storage recommendations
55
Structural formulas   55

DRUGS, EUROPEAN

BT   Drugs
BT   Chemicals, European
NT   Drugs, British
RT   Manufacturers, drugs,
European
Adverse effects 257
Atomic weights 257
Brand names 257
CAS registry numbers 257
Chemical properties 257
Dosage and administration
257
Formulas 257
Molecular weights 257
Pharmacokinetics 257
Pharmacology 257
Physical properties 257
Treatment 257
Uses 257

DRUGS, IMMUNOSUPPRESSIVE

BT   Drugs
Actions and uses 73
Metabolism 73
Pharmacology 73
Toxicology 73

DRUGS, INJECTABLE

BT   Drugs
Compatibility 194

UF–Used For, BT–Broader Term, NT–Narrower Term, RT–Related Term

Concentration   194
Conditional compatibility
194
Dosage and administration
194
Formulation   194
Generic names   194
Incompatibility   194
Manufacturers   194
pH   194
Stability   194
Trade names   194

DRUGS, NEW

BT   Drugs
RT   Investigational drugs
RT   Treatment, experimen-
tal
Acronyms   422
Actions and uses
138
Activities   422
Adverse effects   138
Brand names   138
Composition   422
Descriptions   138
Dosage and administration
138, 422
Equivalents   422
Generic names   422
Indications   138
Investigational code
numbers   422
Manufacturers, drugs   422
Packaging   138
Pharmacokinetics   138
Physical properties   138
Poisoning
Treatment   138
Structures   422
Synonyms   138, 422
Toxicology   138
Trade names   422

DRUGS, NONPRESCRIPTION

UF   Over the counter drugs
BT   Drugs
Actions and uses   349
Adverse effects   349
Brand names   349
Chemical names   349
Dosage and administration
349
Drug interactions   349

Generic names   349
Identification   349
Indications   349
Ingredients   349
Manufacturers, drugs
Addresses   349
Contact persons   349
Telephone numbers   349
Nursing practice
Directions for use   313
Dosage and administa-
tion   313
Formulas   313
Overdosage
Signs and symptoms   349
Treatment   349
Patient education   190

DRUGS OF CHOICE

BT   Drugs
Diseases   15, 139

DRUGS, PRESCRIPTION

BT   Drugs
Adverse effects   348
Brand names   348
Chemical names   348
Dosage and administration
348
Generic names   348
Identifications   348
Illustrations   348
Indications   348
Manufacturers, drugs
Addresses   348
Contact persons   348
Telephone numbers   348

DRUGS (TREATMENT MODALITY)

RT   Drugs
Allergy   12
Communicable diseases
354, 355
Critical care
Nursing practice   295
Diseases   30
Emergency care
Pediatrics   412
Hypertension   78
Newborns   305
Nursing practice   160, 312
Ophthalmology
Pediatrics   336

Oral diseases   5
Patient education   190
Pediatrics   304
Psychiatry   189
Rheumatology   31, 414
Veterinary medicine   435

DRUGS, VETERINARY MEDICINE,
MANUFACTURERS

See Manufacturers, drugs,
veterinary medicine

DUODENUM

BT   Alimentary tract
BT   Gastrointestinal system
Diseases
Treatment, surgical   393

DYING DECLARATIONS

RT   Death and dying
Law
Nursing practice   241

DYING PATIENTS

RT   Death and dying
Family medicine   406

DYSPNEA

Differential diagnosis
244

EAR

See Otolaryngology

EAR DROPS

BT   Drugs
Patient education   280

ECHOCARDIOGRAPHY

BT   Diagnosis
RT   Cardiovascular system
RT   Electrocardiography
RT   Heart
Diseases
Heart   140
Instrumentation   140
Interpretation   140
Techniques   140

ECOLOGY

RT   Air polution
RT   Noise pollution
RT   Radiation pollution
Bacteriology   39

ECONOMIC STATUS

Nursing
Statistical data   157

ECONOMICS

Pharmaceutical practice
371

EDEMA

Differential diagnosis
244

EDITORIAL GUIDELINES

Journals, medical   226

EDUCATION, ALLIED HEALTH
SCIENCES SCHOOLS

See Allied health sciences
schools

EDUCATION, BIOLOGICAL SCI-
ENCES

See Biological sciences
schools

EDUCATION, DENTAL

See Dental schools

EDUCATION, FUNERAL SERVICE
SCHOOLS

See Funeral service schools

EDUCATION, GRADUATE SCHOOLS

See Graduate schools

EDUCATION, HANDICAPPED SPE-
CIAL SCHOOLS

See Handicapped special

schools

EDUCATION, MEDICINE

See Medical schools

EDUCATION, NURSING

RT Nursing schools
Directories 303
Information sources 303
Statistical data 157
  Accreditation 308
  Admissions 308
  Employment information
    308
  Enrollments 308
  Faculties 308
  Graduation 308
  Minority students 308
  Personal information
    308
  Programs 308
  Tuitions 308

EDUCATION, PHARMACOLOGY

See Pharmacy schools

EDUCATION, PUBLIC HEALTH

See Public health schools

EDUCATION, UNDERGRADUATE

See Undergraduate schools

EDUCATION, VETERINARY MEDI-
CINE

See Veterinary medicine
schools

ELDERLY

See Aged

ELECTROCARDIOGRAPHY

BT Diagnosis
RT Cardiovascular system
RT Echocardiography
RT Heart
Interpretations
  Nursing practice 295

ELECTROENCEPHALOGRAPHY

BT Diagnosis
Nervous system
  Encyclopedias, loose-
    leaf 82

ELECTROLYTE DISTURBANCES

RT Acid-base disturbances
RT Body fluid disturbances
RT Diseases
Biochemistry 74
Diagnosis 74, 236, 372,
  392
Nursing practice
  Case histories 314
  Diagnosis, laboratory
    314
  Signs and symptoms 314
Pathogenesis 372
Pathophysiology 74, 236,
  392
Physiology 74, 392
Signs and symptoms 236,
  372, 392
Treatment 74, 236, 372,
  392
Treatment, surgical 110,
  360
  Pediatrics 397

ELECTRONICS

Biology
  Tabular data 96

ELEMENTS

RT Chemistry
Periodic tables 418
Tabular data 95

ELIMINATION

See Pharmacokinetics

EMBRYOLOGY

RT Fetus
RT Growth and development
Atlases 269
Bile ducts 132
Gallbladder 132
Gastrointestinal system
  168, 169

Genitourinary system   57,
172
Genitourinary system,
  female   191
  Anatomy   191
Gynecology   106, 186, 310,
  311, 318
Nomenclature   309
Nursing practice
  Growth and development
  258
  Nervous system   63
  Physiology   258
Obstetrics   310
Ophthalmology   323
Orthopedics   327
Otolaryngology   328

EMERGENCY CARE

UF   First aid
RT   Accidents
RT   Burns
RT   Cardiopulmonary resus-
     citation
RT   Choking
RT   Critical care
RT   High risk patients
RT   Injuries
RT   Intensive care
RT   Poisoning
RT   Toxicology
 Administration   290
 Anesthesia
   Pathophysiology   28
 Cancer   61
 Directories   381
 Diseases
   Assessment, prehospital
   143
   Classification systems
   143
   Diagnosis   142, 143, 290
   Diagnosis, radiologic
   367
   Differential diagnosis
   142
   Etiology   142, 143
   History and physical ex-
     amination   143
   Indications for admis-
     sion   142
   Pathology   142
   Pathophysiology   142,
   143
   Signs and symptoms   143

Stabilization, emergency
  room   143
Treatment   142, 143
Encyclopedias, loose-leaf
  81, 384
Handbooks
  Diagnosis   253, 350
  Signs and symptoms   253
  Treatment   253
Hospital organization   142
Indexes, literature   315
Legal aspects   142
Life support
  Techniques   290
Nervous system trauma
  Pathophysiology   306
  Prognosis   306
  Signs and symptoms   306
  Treatment, surgical   306
Nursing practice
  Assessment   144
  Bites and stings
    Signs and symptoms   144
    Treatment   144
  Joint Commission on Ac-
    creditation
    Requirements
      Interpretations   144
      Standards   144
  Life support   144
  Nursing role   144
  Patient education   144
  Shock treatment
    Assessment   144
    Complications   144
    Etiology   144
    Pathology   144
    Pathophysiology   144
    Signs and symptoms
    144
    Treatment   144
  Trauma
    Assessment   144
    Diagnosis   144
    Signs and symptoms
    144
    Treatment   144
  Triage   144
  Wound treatment   144
Patient education   21
Pediatrics
  Assessment, prehospital
  care   143
  Diagnosis   252
  Differential diagnosis
  412

UF—Used For, BT—Broader Term, NT—Narrower Term, RT—Related Term

Drugs (treatment modal-
  ity) 412
Facility administration
  412
Instructions to parents
  252
Pathophysiology 143,
  412
Resuscitation
  Techniques 412
Signs and symptoms 143,
  192, 252, 412
Stabilization, emergen-
  cy room 143
Treatment 108, 192,
  252, 412
Prehospital transport 142
Sign language 276
Trauma deaths
  Medicolegal investiga-
    tions 292
Triage care 142

ENCYCLOPEDIAS

NT Encyclopedias, loose-
      leaf
RT Dictionaries
RT Handbooks
Allied health sciences
  145
Animals
  Anatomy 146
  Diseases 146
  Genetics 146
  Parasitology 146
  Pregnancy
    Diagnosis 146
  Viruses
    Classification systems
      146
    Nomenclature 146
Bites and stings
  Etiology 196
  Signs and symptoms 196
  Treatment 196
Diseases
  Diagnosis 196
  Etiology 196
  Genetics 196
  Immunology 196
  Pathophysiology 196
  Signs and symptoms 196
  Treatment 196
Ethics, medical 148
Internal medicine 67,

145, 196
Natural ingredients
  Cosmetics
    Chemical composition
      149
    Commercially available
      forms 149
    Pharmacology 149
    Physical descriptions
      149
    Plant sources 149
    Preparation methods
      149
    Synonyms 149
  Drugs
    Chemical composition
      149
    Commercially available
      forms 149
    Pharmacology 149
    Physical descriptions
      149
    Plant sources 149
    Preparation methods
      149
    Synonyms 149
  Food products
    Chemical composition
      149
    Commercially available
      forms 149
    Pharmacology 149
    Physical descriptions
      149
    Plant sources 149
    Preparation methods
      149
    Synonyms 149
Nursing 145
Poisoning
  Signs and symptoms 196
  Treatment 196
Veterinary medicine 146

ENCYCLOPEDIAS, LOOSE-LEAF

BT Encyclopedias
Aged 81
Allergy 81
Cancer 81, 384
Cardiovascular system 81,
  384
Communicable diseases 384
Computed tomography 81
Critical care medicine 81
Dermatology 81, 384

Diagnosis, laboratory   81
Diagnosis, radiologic   81
Diseases
  Classification 81
  Complications 81
  Definitions 81
  Diagnosis 81
  Etiology 81
  History 81
  Incidence 81
  Pathology 81
  Pathophysiology 81
  Signs and symptoms 81
  Treatment 81
Emergency care   81, 384
Endocrine system   81, 384
Environmental medicine
  81
Ethics, medicine   81
Family counseling   81
Family medicine   81
Gastrointestinal system
  81, 384
Genetics 81
Hematology 81, 384
Hospice care   81
Hypertension 81
Immunology 81, 384
Intensive care   384
Internal medicine   384
Kidneys 81, 384
Law 81
Metabolism 81, 384
Nervous system   81, 384
  Aphasias 82
  Cerebral localization
    82
  Cerebrospinal fluid   82
  Computed tomography   82
  Diseases
    Diagnosis 82
    Emotional aspects 82
    Epidemiology 82
    Etiology 82
    Genetic aspects 82
    Pathology 82
    Rehabilitation 82
    Signs and symptoms 82
    Treatment 82
  Drug abuse
    Signs and symptoms 82
    Treatment 82
  Electroencephalography
    82
  Electromyography 82
  Evoked potentials 82

Examination 82
Neuroradiology 82
Neurotoxic agents
  Signs and symptoms   82
Oculomotor systems   82
Psychologic testing   82
Systemic diseases
  Neurologic manifesta-
    tions 82
Visual systems   82
Normal laboratory values
  81
Nutrition 81
Occupational medicine   81
Pharmacology, clinical   81
Physical medicine   81
Preventive medicine   81
Psychiatry 81, 384
Respiratory system   81,
  384
Rheumatology 81, 384
Ultrasonography 81

ENDOCRINE STSTEM

NT   Adrenals
RT   Diabetes
RT   Hormones
RT   Metabolism
RT   Pancreas
RT   Steroids
Anatomy 405
Biochemistry 153, 403
Diseases
  Diagnosis 153, 405
  Etiology 153
  Pathology 405
  Signs and symptoms   153,
    405
  Treatment 153, 405
Encyclopedias, loose-leaf
  81, 384
Genetics 153, 405
Gynecology 310, 311
  Conception 76
  Diseases
    Diagnosis 76
    Physiology 76
    Treatment 76
  Laboratory assays
    Interpretation 76
    Techniques 76
  Obesity 76
  Physiology 76
  Pregnancy 76, 405
  Sexual development   76

Immunology   153
Kidneys   236
Obesity   405
Obstetrics   310, 441
Pathophysiology   153, 331, 388
Physiology   40, 153, 378, 405
Pregnancy   76, 405
Reproduction   153
Sex differentiation   153, 405
Sexuality   89

ENGINEERING

Biology
   Tabular data   96
CRC handbooks
   Indexes   93

ENGINEERING IN MEDICINE

CRC handbooks
   Indexes   93

ENGLISH

Medicine
   Polyglots   141

ENGLISH-SPANISH GLOSSARIES

RT   Dictionaries
Drugs
   Dosage and administra-
      tion   280

ENTOMOLOGIC METHODS

Arthropods
   Parasitology   83
Helminths
   Parasitology   83
Protozoa
   Parasitology   83

ENVIRONMENTAL HEALTH

RT   Air pollution
RT   Industrial hazards
RT   Noise pollution
RT   Occupational health
RT   Radiation pollution
RT   Waste disposal
RT   Water quality manage-
     ment
Encyclopedias, loose-leaf
   81
Public health   259
U.S. government documents
   282

ENZYMES

BT   Proteins
Biochemistry   43, 403
Nomenclature
   Classification numbers
      154
   Names, recommended
      154
   Names, systemic   154
   Reactions   154

EPIDEMIOLOGY (OF DISEASES)

Ambulatory medicine
   358
Cancer   7, 60, 61, 259
Child psychiatry   89
Communicable diseases
   223, 259, 354, 355, 395
   Food poisoning   259
   Nosocomial infections
      259
   Pediatrics   224
   Sexually transmitted
      diseases   259
Dentistry
   Public health   259
Dermatology   26, 116
Gastrointestinal system
   169
Handbooks   104
Heart
   Public health   259
Kidneys   236
   Public health   259
Liver   132
Mental illness   89
   Public health   259
Nervous system   82
Nursing practice   277
Parasitology   83
Pediatrics   339
Rheumatology   31

EPITHELIUM

Atlases
   Histology   33

EQUIPMENT

NT   Hospital equipment
RT   Instruments
RT   Manufacturers, equip-
     ment, medical
Anesthesia   27, 233
Diagnosis, laboratory
   Hematology   207, 240
Nervous system
   Nursing practice   63

EQUIPMENT, MEDICAL, MANUFAC-
TURERS

See Manufacturers, equip-
   ment, medical

ESOPHAGUS

BT   Alimentary tract
RT   Gastrointestinal system
Diseases
   Treatment, surgical   393

ETHICS, MEDICAL

UF   Bioethics
Bibliographies   41
Bibliographies, annotated
   History   246
Codes (text)   148
Encyclopedias   148
Encyclopedias, loose-leaf
   81
Forensic science   292
Indexes, literature   41
Pediatrics   339

ETIOLOGY (OF DISEASES)

RT   Pathogenesis
RT   Pathology
Ambulatory medicine   358
Birth defects   49
Bites and stings   196
Cancer   60, 61
   Statistical data   59
Child psychiatry   89
Chromosomal anomalies   69
Communicable diseases
   223, 355
   Food poisoning   259
   Nosocomial infections
   259
   Public health   259

Sexually transmitted
   diseases   259
Treatment, surgical
   395
Tropical medicine   215
Dermatology   26, 256
Dictionaries   217
Emergency care   142, 143
Encyclopedias   196
Encyclopedias, loose-leaf
   81
Endocrine system   153
Gastrointestinal system
   75, 169
Genetics   270
Genitourinary system   172
Handbooks   67, 104, 286
Hematology   77, 207
Infertility, male   57
Kidneys   236
Laboratory animal sciences
   Handbooks   97
Liver   132, 133
Nervous system   306, 408
   Encyclopedias, loose-
   leaf   82
Neuro-ophthalmology   171
Newborns   382
Nursing practice   242, 277
Ophthalmology   171
Orthopedics   326, 327
   Fractures   327
Otolaryngology   328
Pediatrics   304, 339
   Communicable diseases
   224, 373
   Orthopedics   337
   Poisoning   195
Psychiatry   89
Respiratory system   117,
   365, 413
Rheumatology   31, 414
Sexual dysfunction
   Nursing practice   214
Syndromes   121, 217
Trauma   143
Tropical medicine
   Nutritional deficiencies
   215
   Poisoning
     Fish   215
     Plants   215
Urology   57
Veterinary medicine
   Cats   416
   Cattle   432

UF-Used For, BT-Broader Term, NT-Narrower Term, RT-Related Term

Dogs   416
Horses   432
Pigs   432
Sheep   432
Small animals   113

ETYMOLOGY

NT   Greek etymology
NT   Latin etymology
RT   Terminology
 Bacteriology   39

EUTHANASIA

Death and dying   389
Laboratory animal sciences
 Handbooks   97

EVOKED POTENTIALS

Nervous system
 Encyclopedias, loose-
  leaf   82

EXAMINATION, PHYSICAL

See History and physical
 examination

EXAMINATIONS

UF   Testing procedures
RT   Certification
RT   Licensure
 American Board of Surgery
  415
 Sample questions
  Medical sciences, basic
   Licensure   380
  Medical sciences, clini-
  cal
   Licensure   380
 Testing procedures
  Medical sciences, basic
   Licensure   380
  Medical sciences, clini-
  cal
   Licensure   380

EXCRETION

NT   Urine excretion
RT   Pharmacokinetics
 Biology
  Tabular data   48

Heavy metals
 Toxicology   175
Vitamins   175

EXECUTIVE SEARCH FIRMS

Addresses
 Directories
  Job hunting   362

EXECUTIVES

RT   Administrators
RT   Contact persons
RT   Officials
 Addresses
  Health systems agencies
  184
  Organizations
   Health care business
   184
 Manufacturers, medical de-
 vices
  Catalogs   267
 Multihospital systems
  Directories   184
 Telephone numbers
  Health systems agencies
  184

EXERCISE STRESS

BT   Stress
 Requirements
  Nutrition   293

EXPENSES

NT   Health care expendi-
  tures
RT   Financial aid
RT   Financial data
 Allied health sciences
  schools   341
 Biological sciences
  schools   341
 Dental schools   10, 36,
  341
 Medical schools   36, 275,
  341
 Nursing schools   341
 Pharmacy schools   341
 Public health schools   341
 Veterinary medicine
  schools   341

EXPLOSION DATA

Chemical materials, industrial   114

EYE BANKS

Health care services
Directories   203

EYE DROPS

BT   Drugs
Patient education   280

EYE OINTMENTS

BT   Drugs
Patient education   280

EYES

See Ophthalmology

FACE

RT   Head
Treatment, surgical
Anesthesia   409
Techniques   409

FACILITIES

Dental schools
Directories   36
Hospitals
Directories   184
Medical schools
Directories   36
Research centers
Directories   375
Residency training pro-
grams
Hospitals   178

FACILITY ADMINISTRATION

Emergency care
Pediatrics   412

FAMILIES

Plants, medicinal   247

FAMILY COUNSELING

BT   Counseling services
Encyclopedias, loose-leaf
81

FAMILY MEDICINE

RT   Divorce
RT   Family practice
RT   Internal medicine
RT   Marriage
Adolescence   406
Community resources   406
Diseases
Diagnosis   406
Pathology   406
Signs and symptoms   406
Treatment   406
Dying patients   406
Encyclopedias, loose-leaf
81
Family structure   406
Married couples   406
Patient education   406
Pediatrics   406
Practice management
Computers   406
Financial data   406
Medical records   406
Office design   406
Personnel   406
Single adults   406

FAMILY PLANNING

See Contraception

FAMILY PLANNING CLINICS

Health care services
Directories   203

FAMILY PRACTICE

RT   Family medicine
RT   Practice management
Handbooks
Diseases
Diagnosis   281
Natural history   281
Patient education   281
Prevention   281
Signs and symptoms
281
Treatment   281
Drug abuse   281
Nutrition   281

UF-Used For, BT-Broader Term, NT-Narrower Term, RT-Related Term

Poisoning 281
Sexuality 281

FAMILY STRUCTURE

Family medicine 406
Maternity care
Nursing practice 258

FATIGUE

Differential diagnosis
244

FATTY ACID COMPOSITION

Foods 245
Tabular data 187

FDA CODE NUMBERS

Manufacturers, medical,
devices
Catalogs 267

FEDERAL HEALTH OFFICES

Nursing
Directories 303

FEDERAL INFORMATION CENTERS

Telephone numbers 129

FEDERAL JOB INFORMATION CEN-
TERS

Addresses 129
Telephone numbers 129

FEES

RT Charges
RT Prices
Physicians
Statistical data 363

FERTILITY

RT Infertility
Health
Statistical data 204

FETUS

UF Prenatal care

RT Embryology
RT Obstetrics
RT Pregnancy
Drugs
Adverse effects 296
Genetics
Diseases
Diagnosis 270
Normal laboratory values
232
Obstetrics 191, 305, 441
Monitoring 441
Physiology 318
Treatment, surgical 321

FETUS DEVELOPMENT

Pregnancy
Nursing practice 258

FETUS PHYSIOLOGY

Pregnancy
Nursing practice 258

FEVER

Differential diagnosis
244

FILMS

See Audiovisual materials

FINANCIAL AID

RT Expenses
RT Scholarships
Allied health sciences
schools 13
Dental schools 10, 36
Medical schools 36, 275

FINANCIAL DATA

RT Expenses
Cancer research institutes
Directories 230
Cancer treatment centers
Directories 230
Foundations 163
Hospitals 58, 184
Statistical data 212
Manufacturers, equipment,
medical 263
Manufacturers, products,

medical   263
Organizations   446
Practice management
   Family medicine   406
Research centers   375

FIRES

RT   Burns
RT   Flammability data
Chemical materials,
  industrial
   Control   114
   Hazards   114

FIRST AID

See Emergency care

FISH

BT   Animals, marine
Tropical medicine
   Poisoning (of humans)
      Diagnosis   215
      Etiology   215
      Pathophysiology   215
      Prognosis   215
      Signs and symptoms
      215
      Treatment   215

FLAMMABILITY DATA

RT   Fires
Chemical materials,
  industrial   114

FLAVOR INGREDIENTS

CRC handbooks
   Indexes   93

FLUIDS, BODY

See Body fluids

FLUORIDE

Nutritional content
   Foods   54

FOLACIN CONTENT

Foods
   Tabular data   187

FOOD ADDITIVES

CRC handbooks
   Indexes   93

FOOD CHOICE RECOMMENDATIONS

Diets, modified   187

FOOD-DRUG INTERACTIONS

RT   Drug interactions
Nursing practice   137
   Drugs (treatment modality)
   137

FOOD POISONING

BT   Poisoning
Complications   259
Control   259
Diagnosis   168, 193, 259
Epidemiology   259
Etiology   259
History   259
Immunology   259
Nursing practice   144
Occurrence   259
Pathology   259
Prevention   193, 259
Prognosis   193
Signs and symptoms   168,
  193, 259
Transmission   259
Treatment   168, 193, 259

FOOD PRODUCTS

RT   Foods
Natural ingredients
   Chemical composition
   149
   Commercially available
   forms   149
   Pharmacology   149
   Physical descriptions
   149
   Plant sources   149
   Preparation methods   149
   Synonyms   149

FOOD, SANITARY CONTROL

Public health   259

FOOD SOURCES

UF-Used For, BT-Broader Term, NT-Narrower Term, RT-Related Term

Minerals   296
Vitamins   296
   Handbooks   350

FOOD SUPPLY

   Toxicology
      Chemical additives   293

FOOD VALUES

   Pediatrics
      Tabular data   304

FOODS

   RT   Alcoholic beverages
   RT   Beverages
   RT   Carbohydrates
   RT   Dietetics, clinical
   RT   Diets, modified
   RT   Food products
   RT   Malnutrition
   RT   Minerals
   RT   Nutrition
   RT   Nutritional deficien-
        cies
   RT   Recommended dietary al-
        lowances
   RT   Vitamins
    CRC handbooks
       Indexes   93
    Description   245
    Energy values   245
    Nutritional content
       Amino acids   54, 245
       Cholesterol   54, 187,
        245
       Fatty acids   187, 245
       Fluoride   54
       Folacin   187
       Inorganic constituents
        245
       Iodine   245
       Minerals   54
       Organic acids   245
       Phytic acid   245
       Proximate composition
        54, 245
       Tabular data   170
       Vitamins   54, 245
       Zinc   54, 187
    Poisoning
       Diagnosis   193
       Prevention   193
       Prognosis   193

Signs and symptoms
   193
Treatment   193

FORENSIC DENTISTRY

   BT   Dentistry
   Techniques   292

FORENSIC PATHOLOGISTS

   BT   Physicians
   RT   Pathology
   Directories   381

FORENSIC PSYCHIATRY

   BT   Psychiatry
   Courtroom evidence
      Presentation techniques
       292
   Crime investigations   292

FORENSIC SCIENCE

   UF   Crime
   RT   Courtroom evidence
   RT   Law
   Criminal law investiga-
    tions   292
   Death investigations
    292
   Ethics   292
   History   292
   Medicolegal investigations
      Accidents   292
      Asphyxial deaths   292
      Autopsy techniques   292
      Cause of death determi-
       nation   292
      Courtroom evidence
         Presentation techniques
          292
      Pediatric deaths   292
      Rape   292
      Suicides   292
      Thermal deaths   292
      Time of death determina-
       tion   292
      Trauma deaths   292
   Polygraph technology   292

FORENSIC TOXICOLOGY

   BT   Toxicology
   Medicolegal investiga-

tions 292

FORMULAS

NT   Infant formulas
NT   Molecular formulas
NT   Structural formulas
RT   Ingredients
 Brand names
   Drugs
     Nursing practice   313
 Calculation
   Vital statistics   120
 Commercial products, chem-
   icals 85
 Culture media
   Microbiology   35
 Drugs, European   257
 Drugs, injectable   194
 Media
   Bacteriology
     Diagnosis, laboratory
       179
 Over the counter drugs
   Nursing practice   313
 Pharmaceutical ingredients
   426
 Reagents
   Microbiology   35
 Stains
   Bacteriology
     Diagnosis, laboratory
       179
   Microbiology   35
 Tests
   Microbiology   35

FOUNDATIONS

RT   Grants
 Addresses   164
 Directories   381
   Activities   163
   Addresses   163
   Dates established   163
   Donors   163
   Financial data   163
   Officials   163
   Purposes   163
   Telephone numbers   163
   Trustees   163
 Grants
   Amounts awarded   164
   Application procedures
     163
   Dates authorized   164

 Descriptions   164
 Duration   164
 Limitations   164
 Recipients
   Addresses   164
 Statistical data, aggre-
   gate 163

FOUNTAIN PRODUCTS

 Prices (retail & whole-
   sale)
   Catalogs
     Drug store merchandise
       136

FRACTURE-DISLOCATIONS

 RT   Orthopedics
 Diagnosis   115
 Mechanism of injury   115
 Treatment   115

FRACTURES

 NT   Birth fractures
 RT   Orthopedics
 Anatomy   327
 Classification systems
   165
 Complications   165
 Diagnosis   115, 165
 Diagnosis, radiologic   327
 Dictionaries   254
 Emergency care   136
 Etiology   327
 Historical background
   165
 Mechanism of injury   115
   Pediatrics   337
 Pathogenesis   327
 Pathological anatomy
   165
   Pediatrics   337
 Prognosis   327
 Treatment   115, 165, 327
   Pediatrics   337
 Treatment, surgical   56

FRENCH

 Medicine
   Polyglots   141

FUNERAL INDUSTRY

Licensing requirements
389

FUNERAL SERVICE SCHOOLS

UF Education, funeral ser-
vice schools
Directories
Addresses 389
Programs offered 389
Telephone numbers 389

FUNGI

RT Communicable diseases
RT Mycology
RT Strains, fungi
Laboratory science, clini-
cal
Tabular data 99
Microbiology
Assays 251
Characterization 251
Culture and isolation
251
Examination 251
Identifications 251
Interpretations 251
Serodiagnosis 251
Tests 251
Tabular data 98

GALLBLADDER

RT Bile ducts
RT Biliary ducts, extra-
hepatic
Anatomy 132
Diseases
Diagnosis 132, 133
Pathology 133
Signs and symptoms 132,
133
Treatment 132, 133
Treatment, surgical
Techniques 393
Embryology 132

GASTROINTESTINAL BLEEDING

BT Bleeding
Critical care
Nursing practice 100

GASTROINTESTINAL MANIFESTA-
TIONS

Systemic diseases 168

GASTROINTESTINAL SYSTEM

BT Alimentary tract
NT Anus
NT Colon
NT Duodenum
NT Rectum
NT Stomach
NT Esophagus
Anatomy 168, 169
Diagnostic techniques
168, 169
Diseases
Complications 169
Diagnosis 75, 168, 169
Epidemiology 169
Etiology 75, 169
Incidence 75
Pathogenesis 75
Pathology 75, 169
Pathophysiology 75,
168, 169
Signs and symptoms 75,
168, 169
Treatment 75, 168, 169
Embryology 168, 169
Encyclopedias, loose-leaf
81, 384
Genetics 168
History and physical exam-
ination 168
Immunology 168
Nutrition 169
Pathology 388
Pathophysiology 331
Pediatrics
Diseases
Diagnosis 335
Diagnosis, laboratory
335
Nutritional support
335
Pathogenesis 335
Signs and symptoms
335
Treatment 335
Physiology 168, 169, 378

GENERIC NAMES

UF Names, generic
UF Nonproprietary names
RT Brand names
RT Pharmacological names

RT   Trade names
Drugs   18, 156, 158, 429
  Nursing practice   160
  Patient education   21
  Pediatrics   195
Drugs, injectable   194
Drugs, new   422
Drugs, nonprescription
  349
Drugs, prescription   348
Drugs (treatment modality)
  30

GENETICS

UF   Medical genetics
NT   Cytogenetics
RT   Mendelian inheritance
Abbreviations   9
Acronyms   9
Animals
  Encyclopedias   146
Bacteriology   39
Biochemistry   43
Biology
  Tabular data   48
Chromosomes   270
Counseling   270
  Nursing practice   258
Diseases
  Diagnosis   270
  Diagnosis, laboratory
    287
  Differential diagnosis
    270
  Encyclopedias   196
  Etiology   270
  Fetus
    Diagnosis   270
  Incidence   270
  Metabolism   287
  Modes of inheritance
    368
  Pathogenesis   287
  Pathology   329
  Pathophysiology   287,
    331
  Prognosis   270
  Signs and symptoms   270,
    284
  Treatment   270, 284
Encyclopedias, loose-leaf
  81
Endocrine system   153, 405
Gastrointestinal system
  168

Gynecology   311, 318
Hematology   77
Initialisms   9
Mendelian inheritance
  Bibliographies   284
Mental illness   118
Nervous system
  Encyclopedias, loose-
    leaf   82
Normal variation   270
Obstetrics   318
Pathology   329
Pathophysiology   331
Pediatrics
  Hematology   208
Teratology   270

GENITOURINARY SYSTEM

NT   Genitourinary system,
       female
RT   Abdomen
RT   Urology
Anatomy   57, 172
Diagnostic techniques   172
Diseases
  Complications   172
  Diagnosis   172
  Etiology   172
  Pathogenesis   172
  Prognosis   172
  Signs and symptoms   172
  Treatment   172
Embryology   57, 172
Physiology   57

GENITOURINARY SYSTEM, FEMALE

BT   Genitourinary system
RT   Gynecology
RT   Urology
Anatomy   185
Diseases
  Diagnosis   185
  Signs and symptoms   185
  Treatment   185
Embryology   191
  Anatomy   191
History and physical exam-
  ination   185
Injuries
  Treatment   185
Physiology   191

GERIATRICS

See Aged

GERMAN

Medicine
  Polyglots 141

GLOSSARIES

RT Dictionaries
Chemistry 95
Immunology 37
Mental illness 118
Ophthalmology 316, 323
Otolaryngology
  Nursing practice 316
Physics 95
Psychiatry 89

GOVERNMENTAL AGENCIES

UF Agencies, governmental
UF U.S. government agen-
      cies
RT U.S. government docu-
      ments
Abbreviations 119, 423
Directories
  Abbreviations 423
  Acronyms 423
  Activities 151, 261,
    423
  Addresses 90, 261, 299,
    423
  Directors 261, 299, 423
  Founding dates 151
  History 423
  Information sources 423
  Members, number of 151
  Organizational charts
    423
  Patient education 90
  Staff, number of 151
  Telephone numbers 151,
    261, 299, 423

GRADUATE SCHOOLS

UF Education, graduate
      programs
RT Undergraduate schools
Ratings
  Bacteriology 176
  Biochemistry 176
  Biology 176
  Chemistry 176

Dental schools 176
Medical schools 176
Microbiology 176
Nursing schools 176
Pharmacy schools 176
Public health schools
  176
Toxicology 225

GRANTS

RT Foundations
Activities 261
Addresses 261
Amounts awarded 164
Application procedures
  163
Dates authorized 164
Descriptions 164
Duration 164
Limitations 164
Recipients
  Addresses 164

GREEK COMBINING FORMS

BT Combining forms
RT Latin combining forms
RT Terminology
Health sciences 119
Medicine 119

GREEK ETYMOLOGY

BT Etymology
RT Latin etymology
RT Terminology
Medicine 278
Veterinary medicine 278

GREEK TERMS

BT Terminology
RT Latin terms
Prescription writing 52

GROSS CHARACTERISTICS

Atlases
Diseases
  Pathology, surgical
    8

GROWTH AND DEVELOPMENT

UF Development

NT   Child development
NT   Personality development
RT   Embryology
RT   Growth tables
 Biology
   Tabular data   48
 Dermatology   116
 Hormones
   Endocrine system   405
 Nervous system   359
 Ophthalmology   171
 Pediatrics   108, 192, 304,
 339, 439
   Nursing practice   88
   Tests   195
 Physiology, medical   272

GROWTH TABLES

 RT   Growth and development
 Pediatrics   195

GUIDES

 RT   Handbooks
 RT   Manuals
 Patient education
   Accidents
     First aid   21
   Adolescence   21
   Aged   21
   Anatomy   21
   Childbirth   21
   Contraception   21
   Death and dying   21
   Diseases
     Diagnosis   21
     Prognosis   21
     Signs and symptoms   21
     Treatment   21
   Drugs
     Administration   21
     Adverse effects   21
     Generic names   21
     Trade names   21
   Emergency care
     First aid   21
   Health care system   21
   Infertility   21
   Pregnancy   21
   Sexual disorders   21

GYNECOLOGY

 RT   Abortion
 RT   Childbirth
 RT   Contraception
 RT   Genitourinary system,
       female
 RT   Obstetrics
 RT   Pregnancy
 RT   Reproduction
 RT   Sexuality
 Adolescence   106
   Anatomy   186
   Diseases
     Signs and symptoms   186
     Treatment   186
   Embryology   186
   History and physical ex-
     amination   186
   Physiology   186
   Sexuality   186
 Anatomy   106, 311, 318
   Nursing practice   258
 Cancer
   Treatment, radiation
   318
 Childbirth   106
 Contraception   311
 Cytogenetics   311, 318
 Cytopathology   310
 Diseases
   Classification systems
   191
   Complications   191
   Diagnosis   106, 311, 318
   Differential diagnosis
   191
   Endocrine system   310
   Pathology   191, 310, 311
   Prognosis   191
   Signs and symptoms   106,
   191, 310, 311, 318
   Treatment   106, 191,
   311, 318
   Treatment, surgical
     Complications   401
     Hyperalimentation   401
     Postoperative care
     401
     Preoperative care   401
     Techniques   401
 Embryology   106, 310, 311,
 318
 Endocrine system   311
 Genetics   311, 318
 Histology   310
 History   318
 History and physical exam-
 ination   191
 Pathology

UF–Used For, BT–Broader Term, NT–Narrower Term, RT–Related Term

Abortion   310
Pediatrics   106, 304
  Anatomy   186
  Diseases
    Signs and symptoms
    186
    Treatment   186
  Embryology   186
  History and physical ex-
    amination   186
  Physiology   186
  Sexuality   186
Physiology   76, 106, 311
  Nursing practice   258
Pregnancy   106
Pregnancy, abnormal
  Pathology   310
  Placenta   310
Sex education   311
Sexual response
  Nursing practice   258
Sexuality   106
Treatment, surgical   401
Urology
  Diseases
    Diagnosis   185
    Treatment   185

HANDBOOKS

NT   CRC handbooks
RT   Almanacs
RT   Encyclopedias
RT   Guides
RT   Manuals
Antibiotic drugs
  Adverse effects   105
  Dosage and administra-
    tion   105
  Indications   105
  Pharmacology   105
Antimicrobial drugs
  Adverse effects   105
  Dosage and administra-
    tion   105
  Indications   105
  Pharmacology   105
Biochemistry
  Nomenclature   94
  Tabular data   94
Bites and stings
  Signs and symptoms   111
  Treatment   111
Body surface, adults
  Nomograms   253
Burns

Signs and symptoms   111
Treatment   111
Clinical pharmacology
  Drug prescribing
    Breast feeding   188
    Dietary considerations
    188
    Diseases, drug induced
    188
    Drug interactions   188
    Geriatric drug use
    188
    Immunization schedules
    188
    Nomograms   188
    Parenteral nutrition
    188
    Pharmacogenetics   188
    Pregnancy   188
Communicable diseases
  Diagnosis   354
  Diagnosis, laboratory
    Techniques   354
  Drugs (treatment modali-
    ty)
    Antibiotic drugs
      Actions and uses
      354
      Dosage and adminis-
      tration   354
  Epidemiology   354
  Immunizations
    Adverse effects   354
    Indications   354
    Schedules   354
    Warnings   354
  Nosocomial infections
    354
  Pediatrics
    Diagnosis   373
    Etiology   373
    Immunizations   373
    Treatment   373
  Signs and symptoms   354
  Treatment   354
Dermatology
  Atlases   256
  Classification systems
    256
  Descriptions   256
  Diagnosis   256
  Diagnosis, laboratory
    256
  Differential diagnosis
    256
  Etiology   256

Natural histories   256
Treatment   256
Diagnosis
Techniques   350
Dietetics, clinical   187
Diets, modified
Adverse effects   187
Food choice recommenda-
tions   187
Indications   187
Purposes   187
Diseases
Complications   105
Diagnosis   104, 105,
253, 286
Differential diagnosis
104, 105
Epidemiology   104
Etiology   104, 286
Prevention   286
Prognosis   105, 286
Signs and symptoms   104,
105, 111, 253, 286
Treatment   105, 111,
253, 286
Drugs
Adverse effects   188,
350
Biopharmaceuticals   188
Dosage and administra-
tion   188, 350
Monitoring parameters
188
Patient education   188
Pharmacokinetics   188
Pharmacology   188
Drugs, nonprescription
Diseases
Advice to patient   190
Anatomy   190
Drugs (treatment mo-
dality)
Consumer recommenda-
tions   190
Ingredients   190
Self-medication
guidelines   190
Warnings   190
Etiology   190
Pathophysiology   190
Patient self-diagnosis
190
Physiology   190
Signs and symptoms
190
Emergency care

Diagnosis   253, 350
Signs and symptoms   253
Treatment   253
Family practice
Diseases
Diagnosis   281
Natural history   281
Patient education   281
Prevention   281
Signs and symptoms
281
Treatment   281
Drug abuse   281
Nutrition   281
Poisoning   281
Sexuality   281
Glossaries
Chemistry   95
Physics   95
Immunizations
Administration   253
Adverse effects   253
Recommendations   253
Warnings   253
Laboratory animal sciences
Diseases
Animal hosts   97
Control   97
Etiology   97
Euthanasia   97
Hematology   97
Housing requirements   97
Immunology   97
Legislation   97
Nutrition   97
Organizations
Objectives   97
Physiological data   97
Reproduction   97
Technicians
Training programs   97
Virology   97
Medical schools
Application process   275
Selection process   275
Molecular biology
Nomenclature   94
Tabular data   94
Nervous system
Anatomy   92
Diseases
Diagnosis   92
Differential diagnosis
92
Signs and symptoms   92
History and physical ex-

UF—Used For, BT—Broader Term, NT—Narrower Term, RT—Related Term

amination   92
  Physiology   92
Nomograms
  Body surface area   110
Pediatrics
  Developmental tests   195
  Diseases
    Diagnosis   192, 195,
      439
    Differential diagnosis
      192
    Prognosis   192
    Signs and symptoms
      192, 439
    Treatment   192
  Drugs
    Dosage and administra-
      tion   195
    Generic names   195
    Indications   195
    Trade names   195
    Warnings   195
  Emergency care
    Signs and symptoms
      192
    Treatment   192
  Growth and development
    192, 439
  History and physical ex-
    amination   192
  Nutrition   192
  Poisoning
    Etiology   195
    Signs and symptoms
      192, 195
    Treatment   192, 195
  Psychological tests   195
  Toxicology   439
Poisoning
  Signs and symptoms   111,
    350
  Treatment   111, 350
Psychiatry
  Mental illness
    Drugs (treatment mo-
      dality)
      Complications   189
      Uses and actions
        189
Sign language
  Dentistry   276
  Emergency medicine   276
  Medicine   276
Tabular data
  Algae   98
  Bacteriology   98

Biochemistry
  Amino acids   94
  Buffers   94
  Carbohydrates   94
  Chromatography   94
  Ion exchange   94
  Nucleic acids   94
  Nucleotides   94
  Oligonucleotides   94
  Peptides   94
  Polypeptides   94
  Proteins   94
  Purines   94
  Pyrimidines   94
  Steroids   94
  Vitamins   94
Biology
  Biomechanics   96
  Electronics   96
  Engineering   96
Biomechanics   96
Body composition   170
Body fluids   170
Chemicals   95
Electronics   96
Elements   95
Engineering   96
Food composition   170
Fungi   98
Inorganic compounds   95
Laboratory science,
  clinical
  Bacteriology   99
  Blood banking   99
  Fungi   99
  Hematology   99
  Immunology   99
  Immunopathology   99
  Mycology   99
  Nosocomial infections
    99
  Nuclear medicine   99
  Parasitology   99
  Rickettsiology   99
  Toxicology   99
  Virology   99
Mathematical tables   95
Mathematics   170
Measurement conversion
  tables   95
Microbial composition
  Amino acids   98
  Carbohydrates   98
  Lipids   98
  Minerals   98
  Nucleic acids   98

Proteins 98
Microorganisms 98
Normal laboratory values
  110
Nutrition 170
Organic compounds 95
Physics 95
Probability 170
Protozoa 98
Statistical data 170
Viruses 98
Weights and measures
  110, 170
Travel
  Recommendations 354
Treatment, surgical
  Anesthesia 110
  Body fluids 110
  Communicable diseases
    110
  Complications 110
  Diseases
    Complications 110
    Diagnosis 110
    Prognosis 110
    Signs and symptoms 110
    Treatment 110
  Electrolyte disturbances
    110
  Legal aspects 110
  Metabolism 110
  Nutrition 110
  Postoperative care 110
  Preoperative care 110
  Shock 110
  Transplantation 110
  Wound healing 110
Urology
  Diseases
    Signs and symptoms
      112
    Treatment 112
Vitamins
  Food sources 350
  Nutritional deficiencies
    350
Weight, desirable 110

HANDICAPPED AIDS

  Directories 381

HANDICAPPED SERVICES

  NT Blind services
  NT Deaf services

RT Disability, physical
RT Sign language
RT Speech disorders
  Directories 381

HANDICAPPED SPECIAL SCHOOLS

  UF Education, handicapped
        special schools
  Directories 381

HEAD

  RT Face
  RT Neck
  RT Otolaryngology
  Atlases
    Radiographic anatomy 32
    Surgical techniques 32
  Techniques
    Plastic surgery 411
    Reconstructive surgery
      411

HEADACHE

  Differential diagnosis
    244

HEALTH CARE ADMINISTRATION

  RT Hospital administrators
  Management
    Abbreviations 120
    Acronyms 120
    Dictionaries 120
    Guidelines 197
  Personnel responsibilities
    197

HEALTH CARE BUSINESS

  RT Health care services
  RT Hospitals
  Directories
    Organizations
      Executives
        Addresses 184
        Telephone numbers 184
  Statistical data 199

HEALTH CARE DELIVERY

  Indexes, literature 211

HEALTH CARE EXPENDITURES

UF-Used For, BT-Broader Term, NT-Narrower Term, RT-Related Term

BT   Expenses
  Statistical data   157, 204

HEALTH CARE PRODUCTS, MANU-
FACTURERS, CANADA

  See Manufacturers, health
  care products, Canada

HEALTH CARE RESOURCES

  Utilization
    Statistical data
      Health   204

HEALTH CARE SERVICES

  BT   Services
  RT   Clinics
  RT   Health care business
  RT   Poison control centers
  RT   Runaway youth centers
  RT   Treatment facilities
  Directories
    Administrators
      Addresses   440
      Biographical informa-
        tion   440
      Birth dates   440
      Educational back-
        grounds   440
      Places of birth   440
      Professional back-
        grounds   440
    Adoption   381
    Aged services   203, 381
    Alcoholism treatment
      programs   203
    Architects   381
    Awards   381
    Battered women services
      203
    Blind services   203
    Blood banks   381
    Clinics   203
    Community mental health
      centers   203
    Consulting firms   381
      Addresses   261
      Services   261
      Telephone numbers   261
    Contraception   381
    Coroners   381
    Counseling services   203
    Deaf services   203
    Diagnostic services   203

  Diseases
    Care programs   203
    Organizations   203
    Treatment programs
      203
  Emergency care   381
  Eye banks   203
  Family planning clinics
    203
  Forensic pathologists
    381
  Government health of-
    fices   381
  Grant programs
    Activities   261
    Addresses   261
  Handicapped aids   381
  Handicapped services
    381
  Handicapped special
    schools   381
  Health maintenance or-
    ganizations   381
  Home health agencies
    381
  Hospices   203
  Insurance companies   381
  Laboratories   381
  Legal services   381
  Medical illustrators
    381
  Medical writers   381
  Medicare   381
  Organ transplant regis-
    tries   381
  Pain centers   203
  Pediatric services
    Addresses   297
    Contact persons   297
    Telephone numbers   297
  Public relations   381
  Research centers   381
  Runaway youth programs
    203
  Sex counseling   381
  Sex education   381
  Smoking cessation pro-
    grams   203
  Sudden infant death syn-
    drome centers   203
  Treatment centers   203

HEALTH CARE SYSTEM

  Patient education
    Guides   21

HEALTH FACILITIES

RT   Hospitals
  Inpatients
    Statistical data   199
  Utilization
    Statistical data   157

HEALTH FACILITY ADMINISTRA-
TION

  Indexes, literature   211

HEALTH INSURANCE

  See Insurance companies

HEALTH MAINTENANCE ORGANIZA-
TIONS

  UF   HMO's
  RT   Insurance companies
  Directories   381

HEALTH ORGANIZATIONS

  See Organizations, medical

HEALTH PERSONNEL, WORLD

  UF   Personnel, health,
         world
  Statistical data
    Midwives, number of   443
    Nurses, number of   443
    Physicians, number of
    443

HEALTH PLANNING

  Indexes, literature   211

HEALTH RESEARCH AWARDS

  UF   Research awards, health
  RT   Research programs
  Indexes
    Investigators
      Addresses   374
      Review groups   374
      Subject of projects   374
      Titles of projects   374

HEALTH RISKS

  Medical devices

  Catalogs   267
  Travel   430

HEALTH SCIENCE LIBRARIANSHIP

  RT   Libraries, medical
  Indexes, literature   315

HEALTH SCIENCES LIBRARIES

  See Libraries, medical

HEALTH STATUS

  Secretary of Health & Human Services
    Annual reports   204

HEALTH STATUS DETERMINANTS

  Health
    Statistical data   204

HEALTH SYSTEMS AGENCIES

  RT   Hospitals
  Directories
    Executives
      Addresses   184
      Telephone numbers   184

HEALTHLINE

  BT   Data bases
  RT   Data base access
  Journals
    Abbreviations   243
    History   243
    ISSN's   243
    NLM call numbers   243

HEART

  BT   Cardiovascular system
  RT   Coronary artery dis-
         eases
  RT   Echocardiography
  RT   Electrocardiography
  Anatomy   205
  Diagnostic techniques
  205, 206
  Diseases
    Anesthesia   205, 206
    Complications   206
    Diagnosis   173, 205, 206
    Echocardiography   140

UF-Used For, BT-Broader Term, NT-Narrower Term, RT-Related Term

Epidemiology
  Public health   259
Pathophysiology   205,
  206
Pregnancy   206
Prevention
  Public health   259
Psychiatric aspects   206
Signs and symptoms   205,
  206
Treatment   173, 205, 206
Treatment, surgical   173
History and physical exam-
  ination   205

HEAVY METALS

UF   Metals, heavy
Toxicology
  Chemistry   175
  Diagnosis   175
  Distribution   175
  Excretion   175
  Pharmacokinetics   175
  Sources   175
  Treatment   175

HEIGHT AND WEIGHT TABLES

RT   Weights and measures
Tabular data   187

HELMINTHS

UF   Worms
RT   Parasitology
Biology   83
Classification systems   83
Diagnosis, immunologic   83
Diseases
  Diagnosis   83
  Epidemiology   83
  Pathogenesis   83
  Pathology   83
  Prevention   83
  Prognosis   83
  Signs and symptoms   83
  Treatment   83
Entomologic methods   83
History   83
Illustrations   83
Life cycles   83
Morphology   83
Specimen examination tech-
  niques   83

HEMATOLOGY

RT   Anemia
RT   Arteries
RT   Bleeding
RT   Blood
RT   Cardiovascular system
RT   Circulation
RT   Coagulation factors
RT   Serodiagnosis
RT   Spleen
RT   Thrombosis
RT   Vascular diseases
RT   Veins
Biochemistry   77, 207
Biophysics   77
Cellular biology   77
Cytology   77
Diagnosis, laboratory
  Calculations   207
  Equipment   207
  Interpretations   207
  Interpretations of tests
  179
  Laboratory techniques
  179
  Principles   207
  Purpose   207
  Reagents   207
    Sources   207
  Techniques   207
Diseases
  Diagnosis   77, 207
  Dagnosis, laboratory
    Atlases   240
    Equipment   240
    Normal ranges   240
    Reagents   240
    Techniques   240
  Differential diagnosis
  77
  Etiology   77, 207
  Pathogenesis   77, 207,
  240
  Prognosis   207
  Signs and symptoms   77,
  207, 240
  Treatment   77, 207
Encyclopedias, loose-leaf
  81, 384
Genetics   77
Immunology   77
Laboratory animal sciences
  Handbooks   97
Laboratory science, clini-
cal

Tabular data 99
Molecular biology 77
Pathology
  Physiology 388
Pediatrics
  Blood storage 208
  Blood transfusions 208
  Cell biology 208
  Coagulation factors 208
  Diseases
    Prognosis 208
    Treatment 208
  Genetics 208
  Molecular biology 208
  Normal laboratory values
    208
  Signs and symptoms 208
Physiology 207

HEMOSTASIS

Pathology 330
Treatment, surgical
  Diseases 360

HEPATIC FAILURE

RT Liver
Crisis management
  Nursing practice 100

HIGH RISK PATIENTS

RT Critical care
RT Emergency care
Pregnancy 266

HISTOLOGY

UF Tissues
BT Anatomy
RT Connective tissue
RT Histopathology
Atlases 33
  Diseases
    Pathology, surgical 8
Blood
  Atlases 33
Epithelium
  Atlases 33
Gynecology 310
Integument
  Atlases 33
Mouth
  Diseases 410
Nomenclature 309

Obstetrics 310
Organs
  Atlases 33
Orthopedics 327
Otolaryngology 328
Tissues
  Atlases 33

HISTOPATHOLOGY

BT Pathology
RT Histology
Diseases
  Cats
    Veterinary medicine
    416
  Dermatology 26
  Dogs
    Veterinary medicine
    416

HISTORY

UF History of medicine
RT Medical firsts
RT Original articles
American specialty boards
  126
Animal cell lines
  Cultures
    Catalogs 66
Bibliographies 42,
Biographies 47, 234
Chronologies 234
  Biochemistry 43
Communicable diseases
  Food poisoning 259
  Nosocomial infections
    259
  Public health 259
  Sexually transmitted
    diseases 259
  Tropical medicine 215
Diagnosis, radiologic
  Human body parts 174
Diseases
  Bibliographies 42
  Bibliographies, annotat-
    ed 264
  Encyclopedias, loose-
    leaf 81
  Indexes, literature 42
  Original descriptions
    71
    Physician biographies
    (authors) 71

UF-Used For, BT-Broader Term, NT-Narrower Term, RT-Related Term

Drugs 175
Ethics
  Bibliographies, annotat-
    ed 264
Forensic science 292
Governmental agencies
  423
Gynecology 318
Indexes, literature 42
Nutritional deficiencies
  Tropical medicine 215
Obstetrics 318
Parasitology
  Arthropods 83
  Helminths 83
  Protozoa 83
Physicians
  Biographies 234
Plastic surgery 369
Psychiatry 89, 291
Public health
  Bibliographies, anno-
    tated 264
Toxicology
  Bibliographies, anno-
    tated 264
Treatment, surgical
  Abdomen 4
  Bibliographies 42
  Bibliographies, annotat-
    ed 264
  Indexes, literature 42
U.S. Pharmacopeial Conven-
  tion 426
Vitamins 175

HISTORY AND PHYSICAL EXAMINA-
TION

UF   Examination
UF   Physical examination
RT   Diagnosis
Ambulatory medicine 358
Blood vessels 205
Critical care
  Nursing practice 295
Emergency care 143
Genitourinary system, fe-
  male 185
Gynecology 186, 191, 311
Heart 205
Mouth 324
Nervous system
  Encyclopedias, loose-
    leaf 82
  Handbooks 92

Nursing practice 63
Ophthalmology 171, 323
Otolaryngology 328, 411
Pediatrics 108, 248
  Handbooks 192
  Treatment, surgical
    397
Pelvic examination 311
Respiratory system 117
Rheumatology 84
Techniques 38, 181, 248
Trauma 143
Urology
  Instrumentation 57
  Techniques 57

HISTORY OF MEDICINE

  See History

HMO'S

  See Health maintenance organizations

HOLDINGS (LIBRARIES)

  National Library of Medicine
    Books 302
    Journals 202
    Statistical data 125, 129

HOLISTIC APPROACH

  Critical care
    Nursing practice 100

HOME BIRTH

  BT   Childbirth
  Obstetrics 191

HOME HEALTH AGENCIES

  UF   Agencies, home health
  Directories 381

HORMONE ACTION

  Biochemistry 43

HORMONES

  RT   Adrenals
  RT   Endocrine system
  RT   Steroids

Endocrine system   153
  Aged   405
  Allergy   405
  Dermatology   405
  Growth and development
  405
  Immunology   405
  Metabolism   405

HORSES

  BT   Animals
  Veterinary medicine
  Diseases
    Autopsies   432
    Control   432
    Diagnosis   432
    Etiology   432
    Pathogenesis   432
    Pathology   432
    Signs and symptoms
    432
    Treatment   432

HOSPICE CARE

  RT   Hospitals
  Death and dying   389
  Directories   203
  Encyclopedias, loose-leaf
  81

HOSPITAL ADMINISTRATION

  UF   Administration, hospi-
    tal
  RT   Health care administra-
    tion
  RT   Hospital administrators
  Indexes, literature   211,
  218
  Ordering information
    U.S. government docu-
    ments
      Indexes   282

HOSPITAL ADMINISTRATORS

  BT   Administrators
  RT   Hospital administration
  RT   Management
  Directories
    Addresses   123
    Awards   123
    Birth dates   123
    Birth places   123

Educational backgrounds
123
Marital status   123
Professional backgrounds
123
Telephone numbers   123

HOSPITAL EQUIPMENT

  BT   Equipment
  Directories   381

HOSPITAL ORGANIZATION

  Emergency care   142

HOSPITALS

  BT   Hospitals, world
  NT   Hospitals, Canada
  NT   Hospitals, specialized
  NT   Hospitals, United King-
    dom
  RT   Cancer treatment cen-
    ters
  RT   Clinics
  RT   Health care business
  RT   Health facilities
  RT   Health systems agencies
  RT   Hospice care
  RT   Long-term care
  RT   Multihospital systems
  RT   Nursing homes
  Dental care
    American Dental Associa-
    tion
      Standards   210
    Diagnosis   210
    Emergency dental care
    210
    Infection control   210
    Laboratory service   210
    Medical records   210
    Operating room proce-
    dures   210
    Patient admission   210
    Pediatric patients   210
  Directories
    Accreditation status
    184
    Addresses   184, 261,
    317, 424
    Administrators   184, 424
    Admission statistics
    184, 212
    Bassinets, number of

UF–Used For, BT–Broader Term, NT–Narrower Term, RT–Related Term

184
Beds, number of 128,
  184, 212, 317, 424
Births, number of 184
Census, average daily
  128, 184, 212
Facilities 184
Financial data 184, 212
Financial statistical
  data 184
Nursing
  Employment possibili-
    ties
    Addresses 317
    Beds, number of 317
    Continuing education
      317
    Fringe benefits 317
    Salaries 317
    Telephone numbers
      317
    Working conditions
      317
Occupancy, percentage of
  184, 212
Personnel, number of
  184, 212
Services 212, 424
Telephone numbers 184,
  261, 317, 424
Manuals
Accreditation standards
  6
Quality assurance stan-
  dards
  Diseases
    Charges 332
    Indications for admis-
      sion 332
    Indications for diag-
      nostic tests 332
    Indications for dis-
      charge 332
    Indications for treat-
      ment 332
    Length of stay 332
Residency training pro-
  grams
  Advertisements
    Photographs 178
    Programs offered
      Descriptions 178
      Facilities 178
      Housing 178
      Salaries 178
    Statistical data 178

Statistical data
  Admission statistics
    212
  Beds, number of 212
  Census, average daily
    212
  Financial data 212
  Occupancy, percentage
    212
  Outpatient visits 212
  Payroll 212
  Personnel, number of
    212
  Psychiatric services
    212
  Services 212
  Utilization 212

HOSPITALS, CANADA

  BT Hospitals
  Addresses 58
  Admission statistics 58
  Beds, number of 58
  Births, number of 58
  Department heads 58
  Financial data 58
  Ownership 58
  Telephone numbers 58

HOSPITALS, SPECIALIZED

  BT Hospitals
  Directories 381

HOSPITALS, UNITED KINGDOM

  BT Hospitals
  BT Hospitals, world
  Directories
    Addresses 268
    Beds, number of 268
    Department heads 268
    Telephone numbers 268

HOSPITALS, WORLD

  NT Hospitals
  NT Hospitals, United King-
      dom
  Statistical data
    Admission statistics
      443
    Beds, number of 443
    Discharges, number of
      443

Inpatient days, number of   443

HOUSEHOLD EQUIVALENTS

Tabular data   145

HOUSEHOLD PRODUCTS

RT   Commerical products, chemicals
RT   Cosmetics
RT   Drug store merchandise
RT   Perfumes
Poisoning
Diagnosis   351
Signs and symptoms   351
Treatment   351

HUMAN BODY PARTS

UF   Body parts, human
Diagnosis, radiologic
Anatomy   174
History   174
Physiology   174
Techniques   174

HUMAN BODY SYSTEMS

UF   Body systems, human
Examination
Anatomy   174
History   174
Physiology   174
Techniques   174

HYPERALIMENTATION

RT   Intravenous fluids
Treatment, surgical
Diseases
Gynecology   401

HYPERSENSITIVITY

Immunology   37

HYPERTENSION

RT   Blood pressure
RT   Cardiovascular system
Adolescence   78
Aldosteronism   78
Differential diagnosis 244

Drugs (treatment modality) 78
Encyclopedias, loose-leaf 81
Hypertensive crisis   78
Pathophysiology   78
Pediatrics   78
Pregnancy   78, 266, 372
Renal disease   78
Signs and symptoms   78

IDEAL WEIGHTS

See Weight, desirable

IDENTIFICATION

RT   Atlases
RT   Illustrations
Chemicals, European   155
Color illustrations
Veterinary medicine
Drugs   434
Drugs, nonprescription 349
Drugs, prescription   348
Manufacturers, drugs
Catalogs   19
Microbiology
Bacteriology   251
Fungi   251
Parasitology   251
Pathogenic microorganisms
Atlases   35
Rickettsiae   251
Spirochetes   251
Viruses   251
Pharmaceutical ingredients 426
Procedures
Microbiology
Pathogenic microorganisms   35

IDENTIFICATION TECHNIQUES

Drugs, British   55

IDENTIFICATION TESTS

Drugs   426

ILLUSTRATIONS

RT   Atlases

UF—Used For, BT—Broader Term, NT—Narrower Term, RT—Related Term

RT   Identification
RT   Medical illustrators
Animals, marine   352
Arthropods
  Parasitology   83
Bacteriology
  Indexes   39
Drugs
  Veterinary medicine   434
Drugs, prescription   348
Helminths
  Parasitology   83
Instruments, surgical
  Catalogs   387
Oral manifestations
  Systemic diseases   399
Plants
  Poisoning   353
Poisoning
  Animals, marine   352
Protozoa
  Parasitology   83
Techniques
  Emergency care
    Pediatrics   412

IMMUNIZATIONS

RT   Chemoprophylaxis
RT   Immunology
RT   Prevention
Bites and stings   37
Communicable diseases   37
  Adverse effects   354
  Indications   354
  Schedules   354
  Warnings   354
Diabetes   37
Handbooks
  Administration   253
  Adverse effects   253
  Recommendations   253
  Warnings   253
Pediatrics
  Communicable diseases
    224, 373
  Schedules   108
    Nursing practice   88
  Vaccines   108
  Warnings   108
Rh isoimmunization   37
Schedules   188
Travelers
  Tropical medicine   215
Warnings   296

IMMUNOLOGY

RT   Allergy
RT   Diagnosis, immunologic
RT   Immunizations
RT   Treatment, immunothera-
     py
Allergy   12
Autoimmune diseases
  Immunological tests   250
Autoimmunity   37
Certification   250
Communicable diseases
  Public health   259
Complement   250
Complement system   37
Diagnosis, laboratory
  Interpretations of tests
  179
  Laboratory techniques
  179
  Procedures   37
Diseases   73, 415
  Complications   37
  Diagnosis, immunologic
  37
  Diagnosis, laboratory
  250
  Differential diagnosis
  37
  Encyclopedias   196
  Prevention   37
  Prognosis   37
  Signs and symptoms   37
  Treatment   37
Encyclopedias, loose-leaf
  81, 384
Endocrine system   153
Food poisoning
  Public health   259
Gastrointestinal system
  168
Glossary   37
Hematology   77
Hormones
  Endocrine system   405
Hypersensitivity   37
Immune complexes   250
Immune response   250
Immunoassays   250
Immunodeficiency diseases
  Laboratory diagnosis
  250
Immunogenicity   37
Immunoglobulins   37
Immunohematological tests

250
Infection   37
Laboratory animal sciences
  Handbooks   97
Laboratory science, clini-
  cal
    Tabular data
      Handbooks   99
Licensure 250
Nosocomial infections
  Communicable diseases
    Public health   259
Pathology   329
Pathophysiology   331
Phagocytic cells   37
Reproductive immunity   37
Respiratory system   413
Rheumatology   414
Sexually transmitted dis-
  eases
    Communicable diseases
      Public health   259
Transplantation   37, 360
Transplantation immunology
  Immunological tests   250
Tumor immunology   37
  Immunological tests   250

IMMUNONEPHROLOGY

  Kidneys   236

IMMUNOPATHOLOGY

  BT Pathology
  Communicable diseases   223
  Diseases
    Rheumatology   31
  Laboratory science, clini-
    cal
      Tabular data
        Handbooks   99

IMMUNOSEROLOGICAL TESTS

  Microbiology
    Techniques   251

IMMUNOTHERAPY

  See Treatment, immunotherapy

INCISIONS

  See Treatment, surgical

INCOMES, NET

  RT Salaries
  Physicians
    Statistical data   363

INCOMPATIBILITY

  Drugs   371
  Drugs, injectable   194

INCUBATION PERIODS

  Communicable diseases   91,
    296
  Diseases
    Nursing practice   144
  Pediatrics
    Communicable diseases
      296
  Toxicology
    Food poisoning
      Nursing practice   144

INDEXES

  NT Indexes, literature
  NT Indexes, thesauri
  Bacteriology
    Illustrations   39
  Citations
    Behavioral sciences   383
    Medicine   383
    Science   383
  CRC handbooks
    Analytical toxicology
      93
    Biochemistry   93
    Chemistry   93
    Engineering
      Biology   93
      Medicine   93
    Flavor ingredients   93
    Food additives   93
    Foods   93
    Laboratory animal sci-
      ences   93
    Laboratory safety   93
    Laboratory science   93
    Mathematics   93
    Microbiology   93
    Molecular biology   93
    Nutrition   93
    Physics   93
    Probability   93
    Radioactive nuclides   93

UF-Used For, BT-Broader Term, NT-Narrower Term, RT-Related Term

Scientific tables   93
Statistical data   93
Health research awards
Investigators
Addresses   374
Review groups   374
Subjects of projects 374
Titles of projects   374
Signs and symptoms
Occupational diseases
220

INDEXES, LITERATURE

UF   Periodical literature
indexes
BT   Indexes
RT   Abstracts, literature
RT   Bibliographies
RT   Bibliographies, annota-
ted
RT   Review articles
Allied health sciences
218
Cardiopulmonary technol-
ogy   315
Emergency care   315
Health education   315
Health science librari-
anship   315
Laboratory technology
315
Medical assistants   315
Medical records   315
Medical technology   315
Occupational therapy
315
Physical therapy   315
Radiologic technology
315
Rehabilitation   315
Respiratory therapy   315
Social service   315
Behavioral sciences
Authors
Addresses   383
Bioethics   41
Biography   42
Biomedicine   218
Dentistry   218
Diseases
History   42
Ethics   41
Health care   218
Health care delivery   211
Health facility adminis-

tration   211
Health planning   211
History   42
Hospital administration
211, 218
Medicine
Authors
Addresses   383
Medicine, clinical   218
Medicine, research   218
Nursing   218, 315
Review articles
Behavioral sciences   222
Biomedicine   218
Medicine   222
Medicine, clinical   218
Medicine, research   218
Science and technology
222
Science
Authors
Addresses   383
Teratogenic agents
Chemicals   64
Drugs   64
Physical factors   64
Viruses   64
Treatment, surgical
History   42
U.S. government documents
Ordering information
Behavioral sciences
282
Biomedicine   282
Consumer safety   282
Environmental health
282
Health sciences   282
Hospital administra-
tion   282
Medicine   282
Occupational health
282
Patient education   282
Vital statistics   282
Veterinary medicine   218

INDEXES, THESAURI

BT   Indexes
RT   Thesauri
Core collection
Reference books   162

INDEXING SERVICES

RT   Abstract services
Journals
   Directories   420
Journals, nursing   34

INDICATIONS (DRUGS)

See Actions and uses

INDICATIONS FOR ADMISSION

Diseases
   Emergency care   142
   Hospitals
      Quality assurance
         standards   332

INDICATIONS FOR DIAGNOSTIC
TESTS

Diseases
   Hospitals
      Quality assurance
         standards   332

INDICATIONS FOR DISCHARGE

Diseases
   Hospitals
      Quality assurance
         standards   332

INDICATIONS FOR TREATMENT

Diseases
   Hospitals
      Quality assurance
         standards   332

INDUSTRIAL HAZARDS

RT   Environmental health
RT   Occupational health
RT   Waste disposal
Poisoning
   Diagnosis   351
   Signs and symptoms   351
   Treatment   351

INFANT FORMULAS

BT   Formulas
Tabular data
   Content   187
   Indications for use   187

INFANTS

RT   Newborns
RT   Pediatrics
RT   Sudden infant death
      syndrome centers
Anesthesia   233
   Pathophysiology   28
Nutritional requirements
293

INFECTION CONTROL

RT   Communicable diseases
RT   Nosocomial infections
Critical care
   Nursing practice   295
Hospitals
   Dental care   210
Operating room
   Nursing care   11

INFECTIOUS DISEASES

See Communicable diseases

INFERTILITY

RT   Fertility
Maternity care
   Nursing practice   258
Patient education
   Guides   21
Sexual function, male
   Etiology   57
   Treatment   57
Sexuality
   Nursing practice   214

INFLAMMATION

Pathology   329, 330

INFLAMMATORY PROCESS

Rheumatology   414

INFORMATION CENTERS

RT   Libraries, medical
Directories
   Addresses   129
   Directors   129
   Founding dates   129
   Holdings
      Statistical data   129

UF—Used For, BT—Broader Term, NT—Narrower Term, RT—Related Term

Networks and consortia
  129
Publications 129
Services 129
Special collections 129
Staff names 129
Staff, number of 129
Subjects 129
Telephone numbers 129

Audiovisuals 225
Data bases 225
Graduate schools 225
Legislation 225
Organizations 225
Periodical literature
  225
Reference materials 225
Regulations 225

INFORMATION SERVICES

  RT Libraries, medical
  Directories
    Addresses 150
    Clientele 150
    Directors 150
    Founding dates 150
    Functions 150
    Holdings 150
    Input sources 150
    Publications 150
    Purposes 150
    Services 150
    Staff, number of 150
    Telephone numbers 150

INFORMATION SYSTEMS

  RT Libraries, medical
  Directories
    Addresses 150
    Clientele 150
    Directors 150
    Founding dates 150
    Functions 150
    Holdings 150
    Input sources 150
    Publications 150
    Purposes 150
    Services 150
    Staff, number of 150
    Telephone numbers 150

INFORMATION SOURCES

  RT Bibliographies
  RT Directories
  Allied health education
    schools 13
  Consumer health 90
  Death and dying 389
  Governmental agencies
    Directories 423
  Health care 261
  Medicine 261, 381
  Nursing
    Awards 303
    Clearinghouses, health
      303
    Education 303
    Patient information re-
      sources 303
    Preventive health 303
    Recruitment resources
      303
    Scholarships 303
  Nursing practice 438
  Patient education 90, 145
  Statistical data 390
    Diseases 159
    Health care 159
  Toxicology

INFORMED CONSENT

  RT Patient rights
  Treatment, surgical
    Ophthalmology 322

INGREDIENTS

  NT Natural ingredients
  RT Formulas
  Commercial products, chem-
    icals 85
  Drugs, nonprescription
    190, 349

INITIALISMS

  RT Abbreviations
  RT Acronyms
  Biochemistry 9
  Dentistry 216
  Genetics 9
  Medicine 9, 134
  Pharmacology 9
  Physiology 9
  Science 9

INJURIES

NT   Athletic injuries
RT   Accidents
RT   Emergency care
 Classification systems
  229
 Emergency care
  Diagnosis, radiologic
   367
 Genitourinary tract, fe-
 male
  Treatment   185
 Orthopedics
  Classification systems
   165
  Complications   165
  Diagnosis   165
  Historical background
   165
  Pathological anatomy
   165
  Treatment   165
 Tabular data
  Signs and symptoms   286
  Treatment   286

INORGANIC COMPOUNDS

RT   Organic compounds
 Tabular data   95

INSECT BITES AND STINGS

 See Bites and stings

INSECTICIDES

BT   Chemicals
RT   Pesticides
 Poisoning
  Diagnosis   351
  Signs and symptoms   351
  Treatment   351

INSTRUMENTS

NT   Instruments, surgical
RT   Equipment
 Abbreviations   119
 Dentistry
  Diagnosis   345
 Echocardiography   140
 Urology
  History and physical ex-
   amination   57

INSTRUMENTS, SURGICAL

UF   Surgical instruments
BT   Instruments
RT   Manufacturers, surgical
     instruments
RT   Operating rooms
 Catalogs
  Illustrations   387
  Ordering information
   387
 Nursing practice
  Atlases   228

INSTRUMENTS, SURGICAL, MANU-
FACTURERS

 See Manufacturers, surgical instruments

INSURANCE COMPANIES

RT   Health maintenance or-
     ganizations
 Addresses
  Patient education   90
 Directories   381

INTENSIVE CARE

RT   Critical care
RT   Emergency care
 Anesthesia practice, con-
 sultant
  Techniques   27
 Encyclopedias, loose-leaf
  384
 Pediatrics
  Anesthesia   29

INTERACTIONS

 See Drug interactions

INTERFERENCES

UF   Laboratory test inter-
     ferences
BT   Adverse effects
 Diagnosis, laboratory   20,
  135, 231, 289
  Nursing practice 137,
   239, 312, 313
  Pediatrics   232

INTERNAL MEDICINE

RT   Family medicine

UF-Used For, BT-Broader Term, NT-Narrower Term, RT-Related Term

Dictionaries 67
Encyclopedias 67, 196
Encyclopedias, loose-leaf
  384

INTRAVENOUS FLUIDS

RT Hyperalimentation
Anesthesia 233

INVESTIGATIONAL DRUGS

BT Drugs
RT Cancer protocols, ex-
    perimental
RT Drugs, new
Code numbers 422
Treatment, chemicals
  Cancer 79

IODINE COMPOSITION

Foods 245

ION EXCHANGE

Biochemistry
  Tabular data 94

ITALIAN

Medicine
  Polyglots 141

JAUNDICE

Differential diagnosis
  244

JOB BURNOUT

RT Work stress
Critical care unit person-
nel
  Nursing practice 100

JOB DESCRIPTIONS

Allied health occupations
  13

JOB HUNTING

RT Resumes
Directories
  Executive search firms

Addresses 362
Manuals 362

JOB INTERVIEWING

Career development
  Nursing 317
Manuals 362

JOB TRAINING

Critical care unit personnel
  Nursing practice 100

JOINT COMMISSION ON ACCREDI-
TATION OF HOSPITALS

RT Quality assurance stan-
    dards
Emergency care
  Requirements
    Nursing practice 144
Manuals 6

JOURNALS

UF Periodicals
UF Serials
BT Publications
NT Journals, nursing
NT Journals, United King-
    dom
RT Books
Abbreviations 3, 340
Abstract services   420
Catalogs
  National Library of Med-
    icine
    Bibliographic informa-
      tion 202
    Call numbers 202, 219
    Holdings 202
    ISSN's 202, 219
    Keyword indexes 219
    NLM control numbers
      202, 219
    Subscriptions 202, 219
Clinical practice
Authors
  Addresses 102
Publishers
  Addresses 102
Table of contents 102
Directories
  Abstracting services

420
Addresses 261
Bibliographic informa-
  tion 202, 420
Frequencies 261, 420
Indexing services 420
ISSN's 420
Ordering information
  265, 420
Publishers
  Addresses 265, 420
  Telephone numbers 420
Editorial guidelines 226
Healthline
Bibliographic informa-
  tion
  Abbreviations 243
  History 243
  ISSN's 243
  NLM call numbers 243
Life sciences
Authors
  Addresses 103
Publishers
  Addresses 103
Tables of contents 103
Manuscript preparation
guidelines 226
Medline
Bibliographic informa-
  tion
  Abbreviations 243
  History 243
  ISSN's 243
  NLM call numbers
    243
Popline
Bibliographic informa-
  tion
  Abbreviations 243
  History 243
  ISSN's 243
  NLM call numbers
    243
Proceedings, published
  Journal sources 444
Union lists 202

JOURNALS, NURSING

BT Journals
RT Nursing
Abstracting services 34
Addresses 34
Authors' guides 34
Circulations 34

Frequencies 34
Indexing services 34
Manuscript acceptance cri-
  teria 34
Scopes 34
Subscription prices 34

JOURNALS, UNITED KINGDOM

BT Journals
Addresses 268

KEYWORDS

RT Dictionaries
RT Terminology
Dictionaries 235, 377
Indexes 235, 271, 279
  Journals 219

KIDNEYS

UF Nephrology
UF Renal
RT Cardiorenal system
Acid-bases disturbances
  Diagnosis 236
  Pathophysiology 236
  Signs and symptoms 236
  Treatment 236
Anatomy 236
Diagnosis
  Techniques 372, 392
Diseases
  Diagnosis 236, 392
  Epidemiology 236, 259
  Etiology 236
  Hypertension 78
  Pathogenesis 236, 372
  Pathophysiology 236,
    392
  Physiology 392
  Prevention 259
  Signs and symptoms 236,
    372, 392
  Treatment 236, 372, 392
Electrolyte disturbances
  Diagnosis 236
  Pathophysiology 236
  Signs and symptoms 236
  Treatment 236
Encyclopedias, loose-leaf
  81, 384
Endocrine system 236
Fluid disturbances
  Diagnosis 236

UF-Used For, BT-Broader Term, NT-Narrower Term, RT-Related Term

Pathophysiology 236
Signs and symptoms 236
Treatment 236
Immunonephrology 236
Morphology 392
Pathophysiology 331
Physiology 236
Pregnancy 372
Renal failure
 Pathophysiology 392
 Physiology 392
 Signs and symptoms 236,
  392
 Treatment 236, 392
Renal manifestations
 Systemic diseases 392

KILOCALORIES

Beverages, alcoholic 54

LABOR

See Childbirth

LABORATORIES

RT Diagnosis, laboratory
RT Laboratory service
RT Manufacturers, labora-
     tory equipment
RT Manufacturers, labora-
     tory instruments
 Administration 418
 Directories 381
  Addresses 424
  Services 424
  Telephone numbers 424
 Organization 418

LABORATORY ANIMAL SCIENCES

BT Laboratory science
RT Animals
RT Laboratory science,
     clinical
 Handbooks
  Diseases
   Animal hosts 97
   Control 97
   Etiology 97
   Euthanasia 97
   Hematology 97
   Housing requirements 97
   Immunology 97
   Indexes 93

Legislation 97
Nutrition 97
Organizations
 Objectives 97
 Physiological data 97
 Reproduction 97
Technicians
 Training programs 97
Virology 97

LABORATORY DIAGNOSIS

See Diagnosis, laboratory

LABORATORY EQUIPMENT MANUFAC-
TURERS

See Manufacturers, laboratory equipment

LABORATORY INSTRUMENTS, MANU-
FACTURERS

See Manufacturers, laboratory instruments

LABORATORY SAFETY

CRC handbooks
 Indexes 93

LABORATORY SCIENCE

NT Laboratory animal sci-
     ences
NT Laboratory science,
     clinical
 CRC handbooks
  Indexes 93

LABORATORY SCIENCE, CLINICAL

BT Laboratory science
RT Chemistry
RT Laboratory animal sci-
     ences
RT Reagents
 Tabular data
  Bacteriology 99
  Blood banking 99
  Fungi 99
  Hematology 99
  Immunology 99
  Immunopathology 99
  Mycology 99
  Nosocomial infections

99
Nuclear medicine   99
Parasitology   99
Rickettsiology   99
Toxicology   99
Virology   99

LABORATORY SERVICE

RT   Laboratories
Classification systems
347
Hospitals
Dental care   210

LABORATORY TECHNIQUES

RT   Assays
RT   Diagnosis, laboratory
Abbreviations   3
Classification systems
347
Clinical chemistry   179
Hematology   179
Immunology   179
Microbiology   35
Mycology   179
Parasitology   179
Serology   179

LABORATORY TECHNOLOGY

Indexes, literature   315

LABORATORY TEST INTERFERENCES

See Interferences

LABORATORY VALUES

See Normal laboratory
values

LACTATION

See Breast feeding

LATIN COMBINING FORMS

BT   Combining forms
RT   Greek combining forms
RT   Terminology
Health sciences   119
Medicine   119

LATIN ETYMOLOGY

BT   Etymology
RT   Greek etymology
RT   Terminology
Terminology
Medicine   278
Veterinary medicine   278

LATIN TERMS

RT   Greek terms
RT   Terminology
Medical orders
Abbreviations
Nursing practice   313
Prescription writing   52,
391

LAW

UF   Crime
RT   Courtroom evidence
RT   Forensic science
RT   Medicolegal investiga-
tions
RT   Patient rights
Abortion, induced   191
Death and dying   389
Emergency care   142
Encyclopedias, loose-leaf
81
Nursing practice   241
Critical care unit per-
sonnel   100
Dying declarations   241
Liabilities   241
Licensure   241
Malpractice   241
Negligence   241
Professional responsi-
bilities   241
Torts   241
U.S. court system   241
U.S. governmental struc-
ture   241
U.S. jurisprudence   241
U.S. legislation   241
Wills   241
Witnesses   241
Pediatrics
Anesthesia   29
Psychiatry   291
Treatment, surgical   110

LEGAL SERVICES

Directories   381

UF–Used For, BT–Broader Term, NT–Narrower Term, RT–Related Term

LEGISLATION

    Laboratory animal sciences
    97
    Pharmaceutical practice
    371
    Toxicology
      Information sources 225

LENGTH OF STAY

    Diseases
      Hospitals
        Quality assurance
        standards 332

LIBRARIES FOR THE BLIND

    Addresses 129, 261
    Directors 129
    Telephone numbers 129,
    261

LIBRARIES, MEDICAL

    UF   Health sciences librar-
        ies
    BT   Libraries, special
    NT   National Library of
        Medicine
    RT   Health science librar-
        ianship
    RT   Information centers
    RT   Information systems
    Addresses 125, 261
    Data base access 125
    Directors 125, 261
    Holdings
      Statistical data 125,
      261
    Personnel
      Statistical data 125
    Sponsoring organizations
    125
    Telephone numbers 261

LIBRARIES, RESEARCH

    UF   Research libraries
    Directories
      Addresses 129
      Directors 129
      Founding dates 129
      Holdings 129
      Networks and consortia
      129

      Publications 129
      Services 129
      Special collections 129
      Staff names 129
      Staff, number of 129
      Telephone numbers 129

LIBRARIES, RESEARCH CENTERS

    RT   Research centers
    Directories 375

LIBRARIES, SPECIAL

    UF   Special libraries
    NT   Libraries, medical
    RT   Archives
    Addresses 129
    Directors 129
    Founding dates 129
    Holdings 129
    Networks and consortia
    129
    Publications 129
    Services 129
    Special collections 129
    Staff names 129
    Staff, number of 129
    Telephone numbers 129

LIBRARIES, WORLD

    Addresses 445
    Directors 445
    Holdings 445

LIBRARY NETWORKS

    Directories
      Addresses 129
      Directors 129
      Telephone numbers 129

LICENSURE

    NT   Dental licensure
    RT   Certification
    RT   Examinations
    Foreign requirements 442
    Funeral industry require-
    ments 389
    Immunology requirements
    250
    Manpower
      Statistical data 199
    Medical sciences

Examination boards,
state
  Addresses 424
  Telephone numbers 424
Examinations
  Sample questions 380
  Testing procedures
  380
National requirements
425
State requirements 128,
425
Statistical data 425
Nursing practice 241, 303

LIFE SUPPORT

See Critical care

LIFE TABLES

UF Actuarial tables
Tabular data 437

LIPIDS

RT Nutrition
Biosynthesis
  Biochemistry 43
Microbial composition
  Tabular data 98

LIVER

RT Bile ducts
RT Hepatic failure
Anatomy 132, 133
Biochemistry 132
Diagnostic techniques 132
Diseases
  Diagnosis 132, 133
  Epidemiology 132
  Etiology 132, 133
  Pathology 132, 133
  Prognosis 133
  Signs and symptoms 132,
  133
  Treatment 132, 133
  Treatment, surgical
    Techniques 393
Metabolism 132
Pathophysiology 331
Physiology 132
Transplantation
  Indications 132
  Techniques 132

LONG-TERM CARE

RT Hospitals
Aged 72

LUNGS

See Respiratory system

LYMPH

Body fluids
  Physiology 40

MALARIA RISKS

Travel 430

MALNUTRITION

RT Foods
RT Nutrition
RT Nutritional deficien-
    cies
Diagnosis, radiologic 293
Differential diagnosis
244
Obesity 293
Signs and symptoms 293
Treatment 293
Vitamin analysis 293

MANAGEMENT

RT Hospital administra-
    tion
Abbreviations 120
Acronyms 120
Dictionaries 120
Guidelines 197

MANIFESTATIONS OF SYSTEMIC
DISEASES

See Systemic diseases

MANUALS

RT Guides
RT Handbooks
Copy editing marks 249
Hospitals
  Accreditation standards
  6
Job hunting 362
Job interviewing 362

UF—Used For, BT—Broader Term, NT—Narrower Term, RT—Related Term

Nursing practice
  Diagnosis
    Techniques 242
  Treatment
    Techniques 242
Proofreading marks 249
Publishing, medical 213
Resumes 362
Terminology 447
Writing, medical 213

MANUFACTURERS, CHEMICALS

  UF Chemical manufacturers
  RT Chemicals
  Addresses 68, 85
  Telephone numbers 68, 85
  Telex numbers 68
  Tollfree telephone numbers
    68
  TWX numbers 68

MANUFACTURERS, DRUGS

  UF Drug manufacturers
  UF Pharmaceutical compa-
      nies
  NT Manufacturers, drugs,
      European
  NT Manufacturers, drugs,
      veterinary medicine
  RT Drugs
  Directories 381
    Addresses 18, 19, 136,
      348, 349
    Calandars, merchandising
      136
    Catalogs 19, 136
    Contact persons 348,
      349
    Identification 19
    National drug code num-
      bers 19
    Packaging 19
    Prices 19
    Return policies 136
    Telephone numbers 136,
      348, 349
  Packaging 371
  Preformulations 371
  Sterilization 371

MANUFACTURERS, DRUGS, EURO-
PEAN

  UF Drugs, European, manu-

      facturers
  BT Manufacturers, drugs
  RT Chemicals, European
  RT Drugs, British
  RT Drugs, European
  Addresses 257

MANUFACTURERS, DRUGS, VETER-
INARY MEDICINE

  UF Drugs, veterinary med-
      icine, manufacturers
  BT Manufacturers, drugs
  RT Drugs
  Addresses 434

MANUFACTURERS, EQUIPMENT,
MEDICAL

  UF Equipment, medical,
      manufacturers
  RT Equipment
  Directories
    Addresses 263
    Distributors 263
    Employees, number of
      263
    Financial data 263
    Officials 263
    Sales statistics 263
    Telephone numbers 263

MANUFACTURERS, HEALTH CARE
PRODUCTS, CANADA

  UF Health care products,
      manufacturers, Canada
  Buyers' guides
    Addresses 58
    Contact persons 58
    Telephone numbers 58

MANUFACTURERS, LABORATORY
EQUIPMENT

  UF Laboratory equipment
      manufacturers
  RT Laboratories
  Directories
    Addresses 183
    Telephone numbers 183

MANUFACTURERS, LABORATORY
INSTRUMENTS

  UF Laboratory instruments,

manufacturers
RT   Laboratories
Directories
   Addresses   183
   Telephone numbers   183

MANUFACTURERS, MEDICAL DE-
VICES

UF   Medical device manu-
     facturers
Catalogs
   Addresses   267
   Distributors   267
   Employees, number of
     267
   Executives   267
   FDA code numbers   267
   Health risks   267
   Local dealers   267
   Ownership   267
   Prices   267
   Regulations   267
   Standards   267
   Telephone numbers   267

MANUFACTURERS, MEDICAL PRO-
DUCTS

UF   Medical products,
     manufacturers
Directories
   Addresses   263
   Distributors   263
   Employees, number of
     263
   Financial data   263
   Officials   263
   Sales statistics   263
   Telephone numbers   263

MANUFACTURERS, SURGICAL IN-
STRUMENTS

UF   Instruments, surgical,
     manufacturers
UF   Surgical instruments,
     manufacturers
RT   Instruments, surgical
Catalogs
   Addresses   387
   Illustrations   387
   Ordering information
     387
   Telephone numbers   387

MANUSCRIPT ACCEPTANCE CRITE-
RIA

Journals, nursing   34

MANUSCRIPT PREPARATION

Guidelines   226
Publishing, medical   213
   Style manuals   249
Writing, medical   213

MARRIAGE

RT   Divorces
RT   Family medicine
   Statistical data   436, 437

MATHEMATICAL CONSTANTS

Biology
   Tabular data   48

MATHEMATICS

RT   Weights and measures
CRC handbooks
   Indexes   93
   Tabular data   95, 170

MAXILLA

RT   Dentistry, operative
Treatment, surgical
   Anesthesia   409
   Techniques   409

MEASUREMENT

See Weights and measures

MEDIA

Formulas
   Diagnosis, laboratory
      Bacteriology   179

MEDIC ALERT

Directories   203

MEDICAL ASSISTANTS

Allied health sciences
   Indexes, literature   315

MEDICAL DEVICE MANUFACTURERS

See Manufacturers, medical devices

MEDICAL EDUCATION

See Medical schools

MEDICAL FIRSTS

RT   History
RT   Original articles
  Bibliographies
    Diagnostic techniques 152
    Diseases   152
    Strains   152
    Surgical techniques   152

MEDICAL GENETICS

See Genetics

MEDICAL ILLUSTRATORS

RT   Illustrations
  Directories   381

MEDICAL ORDERS

  Abbreviations   18
  Latin terms
    Nursing practice
      Abbreviations   313

MEDICAL PRODUCTS, MANUFAC-
TURERS

See Manufacturers, medical products

MEDICAL RECORDS

NT   Problem-oriented medi-
     cal records
  Allied health sciences
    Indexes, literature   315
  Data elements   332
  Hospitals
    Dental care   210
  Nursing practice
    Interpretation   167
  Practice management
    Family medicine   406

MEDICAL SCHOOLS

UF   Medical education
BT   University programs
NT   Medical schools, for-
     eign
RT   Association of American
     Medical Colleges
RT   Medical schools, United
     Kingdom
RT   Premedical programs
RT   Residency programs, ac-
     credited
  Application process   275
  Directories
    Academic calendars   1,
    275
    Addresses   1, 2, 36,
    261, 275, 424
    Admission requirements
    36, 275
    Admission statistics   36
    Clinical facilities   2
    Curricula   1, 36, 275
    Deans   261
    Enrollment data   2
    Expenses   36, 275
    Facilities   2, 36
    Financial aid   36, 275
    Founding dates   2
    Officials   2, 275
    Selection factors   275
    Statistical data   275
    Telephone numbers   1, 2,
    261, 275
  Ratings
    Graduate schools   176
  Selection process   275

MEDICAL SCHOOLS, FOREIGN

BT   Medical schools
BT   Universities, world
BT   University programs
NT   Medical schools, United
     Kingdom
  Directories
    Addresses   36, 261, 442
    Admission requirements
    36
    Admission statistics
    442
    Enrollment, number of
    442
    Faculty, number of   442
    Founding dates   442

Graduates, number of
442
Language of instruction
442

MEDICAL SCHOOLS, UNITED KING-
DOM

BT Medical schools, for-
eign
RT Medical schools
Directories
Addresses 268
Administrators 268
Department heads 268
Telephone numbers 268

MEDICAL SPECIALISTS

See American specialty
boards

MEDICAL TERMINOLOGY

See Terminology

MEDICARE

Directories 381

MEDICOLEGAL INVESTIGATIONS

RT Law
Accidents 292
Asphyxial deaths 292
Autopsy techniques
292
Cause of death deter-
mination 292
Courtroom evidence
Presentation tech-
niques 292
Pediatric deaths 292
Rape 292
Suicides 292
Thermal deaths 292
Time of death determina-
tion 292
Trauma deaths 292

MEDLINE

BT Data bases
RT Data base access
Journals
Abbreviations 243

History 243
ISSN's 243
NLM call numbers 243

MEETINGS, FUTURE

UF Conferences
UF Conventions
RT Meetings, past
Directories
Attendees, estimated
number of 444
Contact persons 386,
444
Dates 386, 444
Exhibit information 444
Languages 444
Locations 386, 444
Paper submission dead-
lines 444
Proceedings, sources of
444
Sponsors 386, 444
Subject content 444
Translation facilities
444

MEETINGS, PAST

UF Conferences
UF Conventions
RT Meetings, future
RT Proceedings, published
Dates 127, 221
Locations 127, 221
Sponsors 127, 221

MEMBERSHIP

American College of Physi-
cians 45
American College of Sur-
geons 16
American Dental Associa-
tion 17
American Hospital Associa-
tion 184
American Psychiatry Asso-
ciation 44
American Public Health As-
sociation 46
American specialty boards
126
Association of American
Medical Colleges 2
Congressional subcommit-

UF-Used For, BT-Broader Term, NT-Narrower Term, RT-Related Term

tees 299
Council on Dental Thera-
  peutics 5
Governmental agencies
  Statistical data 151
Organizations, dental
  Statistical data 151
Organizations, medical
  Statistical data 147,
  151, 198, 261, 446
Organizations, nursing
  Statistical data 151
Organizations, pharmaco-
  logy
  Statistical data 151

MENDELIAN INHERITANCE

RT Genetics
Birth defects 49
Diseases
  Bibliographies 284
  Dictionaries 217
  Signs and symptoms
  284
  Synonyms 217, 284

MENTAL HEALTH

Thesauri 262

MENTAL HEALTH SERVICES

NT Counseling services
Pediatrics
  Addresses 297
  Contact persons 297
  Telephone numbers 297

MENTAL ILLNESS

RT Child psychiatry
RT Community mental health
    centers
RT Counseling services
RT Diseases
RT Psychiatry
Age at onset 118
Case studies 291
Classification systems
  118
Complications 118
Diagnosis 291
Differential diagnosis
  Decision trees 118
Drugs (treatment modality)

89, 189, 291
  Complications 189
  Actions and uses 189
Genetics 118
Glossaries 118
History and physical exam-
  ination 181
Natural history 118
Nomenclature 118
Predisposing factors 118
Prevalence 118
Public health
  Epidemiology 259
  Prevention 259
Sex ratio 118
Signs and symptoms 118,
  291
Treatment 291

MENTAL RETARDATION

Psychiatry 291
Public health
  Epidemiology 259
  Prevention 259

METABOLISM

NT Catabolism
RT Digestion
RT Endocrine system
Biochemistry 403
Biology
  Tabular data 48
Birth defects 49, 287
Cardiovascular drugs
  Nursing practice 62
Control mechanisms 288
Diseases 217, 287, 288
  Modes of inheritance
  368
Drugs, immunosuppressive
  73
Encyclopedias, loose-leaf
  81, 384
Hormones
  Endocrine system 405
Liver 132
Minerals
  Nutrition 293
Pathology
  Physiology 388
Pathophysiology 331
Physiology 272, 378
Rheumatology 414
Syndromes 217

Vitamins
    Nutrition 298

METALS, HEAVY

    See Heavy metals

MICROBIAL COMPOSITION

    Tabular data
        Amino acids   98
        Carbohydrates   98
        Lipids 98
        Minerals 98
        Nucleic acids   98
        Proteins 98

MICROBIOLOGY

    NT   Bacteriology
    RT   Stains
    Clinical specimen proce-
      dures 35
    Communicable diseases
      Treatment, surgical   395
    Culture media
        Formulas 35
        Procedures 35
    CRC handbooks
        Indexes 93
    Fungi
        Assays 251
        Characterization 251
        Culture and isolation
          251
        Examination 251
        Identification 251
        Interpretations 251
        Serodiagnosis 251
        Tests 251
    Graduate schools
        Ratings 176
    Immunoserological tests
        Techniques 251
    Laboratory procedures   35
    Otolaryngology 328
    Parasitology
        Assays 251
        Characterization 251
        Culture and isolation
          251
        Examination 251
        Identification 251
        Interpretations 251
        Serodiagnosis 251
        Tests 251

Pathogenic microorganisms
    Cultivation 35
    Diagnosis
        Serologic procedures
          35
    Identification
        Atlases 35
        Procedures 35
    Reagents
        Formulas 35
        Procedures 35
    Rickettsiae
        Assays 251
        Characterization 251
        Culture and isolation
          251
        Examination 251
        Identification 251
        Interpretations 251
        Serodiagnosis 251
        Tests 251
    Spirochetes
        Assays 251
        Characterization 251
        Culture and isolation
          251
        Examination 251
        Identification 251
        Interpretations 251
        Serodiagnosis 251
        Tests 251
    Stains
        Formulas 35
        Procedures 35
    Tests
        Formulas 35
        Procedures 35
    Undergraduate schools   177
    Viruses
        Assays 251
        Characterization 251
        Culture and isolation
          251
        Examination 251
        Identification 251
        Interpretations 251
        Serodiagnosis 251
        Tests 251

MICROORGANISMS

    Tabular data 98

MIDWIVES, NUMBER OF

    RT   Childbirth

Health personnel, world
    Statistical data   443

MIGRANT HEALTH CENTERS

    Directories   203

MINERALS

    RT   Foods
    RT   Nutrition
    Food sources   296
    Microbial composition
        Tabular data   98
    Nutrition
        Metabolism   293
        Requirements   293
    Nutritional content
        Foods   54
    Nutritional deficiencies
    293, 296
    Physiological functions
    296
    Requirements   296

MINORITY STUDENTS

    Statistical data
        Education, nursing   308

MOLECULAR BIOLOGY

    BT   Biology
    CRC handbooks
        Indexes   93
    Hematology   77
        Pediatrics   208
    Nomenclature   94
    Tabular data   94

MOLECULAR FORMULAS

    BT   Formulas
    Chemicals   285, 370
    Chemicals, European   155
    Drugs   285, 371, 426, 429
    Drugs, British   55

MOLECULAR WEIGHTS

    BT   Weights and measures
    Chemicals   285, 370
    Drugs   285, 429
    Drugs, European   257

MORBIDITY

    RT   Mortality
    RT   Vital statistics
    Communicable diseases
        Statistical data
            Ages   443
            Seasonal distributions
            443
            Sexes   443

MORPHOLOGY

    RT   Anatomy
    Diseases   329
    Kidneys   392
    Neoplasms
        Classification systems
        229
    Parasitology
        Arthropods   83
        Helminths   83
        Protozoa   83
    Pathology
        Classification systems
        398
    Respiratory system   413

MORTALITY

    UF   Death rate
    NT   Mortality, fetal
    NT   Mortality, infant
    RT   Death and dying
    RT   Morbidity
    RT   Suicides
    Statistical data   204, 436
        Accidents   437
        Ages of death   443
        Cancer   59
        Causes of death   437
        Characteristics   437
        Rates   437
        Sexes   443

MORTALITY, FETAL

    BT   Mortality
    Statistical data
        Causes of death   437
        Characteristics   437
        Rates   437

MORTALITY, INFANTS

    BT   Mortality
    Statistical data
        Causes of death   437,

443
Characteristics   437
Rates   437

MOTILE SYSTEM

Biochemistry   43

MOTOR FUNCTIONS

Neurophysiology
Disability, physical
237

MOUTH

BT   Alimentary tract
RT   Dentistry
RT   Oral diseases
RT   Oral manifestations
Diseases
Examination techniques
324
Histology   410
Prognosis   410
Signs and symptoms   324,
410
Treatment   324, 410
Treatment, surgical
393, 409

MULTIHOSPITAL SYSTEMS

RT   Hospitals
Directories
Addresses   184
Executives   184
Telephone numbers   184

MUSCLES

RT   Orthopedics
Anatomical tables   52,
145, 283
Biochemistry   43

MUSEUMS, WORLD

Directories
Addresses   445
Directors   445
Holdings   445

MYCOLOGY

RT   Communicable diseases

RT   Fungi
RT   Strains, fungi
Diagnosis, laboratory
Interpretations of tests
179
Laboratory techniques   179
Laboratory science, clini-
cal
Tabular data   99

MYCOVIRUSES

See Strains, mycoviruses

NAME CHANGES

Drugs   18

NAMES, ACCEPTED

Bacteriology
Etymologies   39

NAMES, BRAND

See Brand names

NAMES, CHEMICAL

See Chemical names

NAMES, GENERIC

See Generic names

NAMES, NONPROPRIETARY

See Generic names

NAMES, PHARMACOLOGICAL

See Pharmacological names

NAMES, PROPRIETARY

See Brand names

NAMES, RECOMMENDED

Enzymes
Nomenclature   154

NAMES, SCIENTIFIC

See Scientific names

UF—Used For, BT—Broader Term, NT—Narrower Term, RT—Related Term

NAMES, SYSTEMIC

  Enzymes
    Nomenclature   154

NAMES, TRADE

  See Trade names

NATALITY

  RT Births, number of
  RT Vital statistics
    Statistical data   436
      Characteristics   437
      Rates   437

NATIONAL DRUG CODES

  Drugs   19, 298

NATIONAL LIBRARY OF MEDICINE

  BT Libraries, medical
    Catalogs
      Audiovisual materials
        Bibliographic informa-
          tion   300
        Ordering information
          300
        Reviews   300
      Books
        Bibliographic infor-
          mation   302
        Call numbers   302
      Journals
        Bibliographic infor-
          mation   202
        Call numbers   202, 219
        Holdings   202
        ISSN's   202, 219
        Keyword indexes   219
        NLM control numbers
          202, 219
        Subscriptions   202,
          219

NATURAL INGREDIENTS

  BT Ingredients
    Encyclopedias
      Cosmetics
        Chemical composition
          149
        Commercially available
          forms   149

        Pharmacology   149
        Physical descriptions
          149
        Plant sources   149
        Preparation methods
          149
        Synonyms   149
      Drugs
        Chemical composition
          149
        Commercially available
          forms   149
        Pharmacology   149
        Physical descriptions
          149
        Plant sources   149
        Preparation methods
          149
        Synonyms   149
      Food products
        Chemical composition
          149
        Commercially available
          forms   149
        Pharmacology   149
        Physical descriptions
          149
        Plant sources   149
        Preparation methods
          149
        Synonyms   149

NAUSEA

  Differential diagnosis
    244

NECK

  RT Head
  RT Otolaryngology
    Atlases
      Radiographic anatomy
        32
    Techniques
      Plastic surgery   411
      Reconstructive surgery
        411
    Treatment, surgical   32

NECROPSIES

  See Autopsies

NEOPLASMS

See Cancer

NEPHROLOGY

See Kidneys

NERVES

Anatomical tables   52,
145, 283

NERVOUS SYSTEM

UF   Central nervous system
UF   Neurology
UF   Neurosurgery
RT   Neurobiology
RT   Neurologic manifesta-
     tions
RT   Neuro-ophthalmology
RT   Neurophysiology
RT   Neuroradiology
Anatomy   92, 359
Anesthesia   233
Diagnosis
   Techniques   92, 306, 359
Diseases
   Diagnosis   82, 92, 306,
   408
   Diagnosis, radiologic
   82
   Differential diagnosis
   92, 359
   Epidemiology   82
   Etiology   82, 306, 408
   Genetics   82
   History and physical ex-
   amination   82, 92
   Incidence   408
   Pathogenesis   306
   Pathology   82, 408
   Prognosis   306
   Rehabilitation   82
   Signs and symptoms   82,
   92, 359, 408
   Treatment   82, 306, 408
   Treatment, surgical
   Techniques   306
Drug abuse
   Signs and symptoms   82
   Treatment   82
Encyclopedias, loose-leaf
   81, 82, 384
Evoked potentials   82
Growth and development
   359

Human behavior   89
Nursing practice
   Anatomy   63
   Diseases
      Classification   63
      Diagnosis   63
      Nursing intervention
      63
      Prognosis   63
   Embryology   63
   Equipment   63
   History and physical ex-
   amination   63
      Newborns   258
   Physiology   63
   Standards of care   63
Oculomotor systems   82
Pain
   Physiology   306
   Treatment   306
Pathophysiology   331
Physiology   40, 92, 272,
306, 378
Psychologic testing   82
Trauma
   Pathophysiology   306
   Prognosis   306
   Signs and symptoms   306
   Treatment, surgical
   Techniques   306
Visual systems   82

NERVOUSNESS

Differential diagnosis
244

NEUROBIOLOGY

RT   Nervous system
Biology
   Tabular data   48

NEUROLOGIC MANIFESTATIONS

RT   Nervous system
Systemic diseases
   Encyclopedias, loose-
   leaf   82

NEUROLOGY

See Nervous system

NEURO-OPHTHALMOLOGY

BT   Ophthalmology
RT   Nervous syetem
Diseases
  Etiology 171
  Signs and symptoms 171

NEUROPHYSIOLOGY

BT   Physiology
RT   Nervous system
Disability, physical
  Motor functions   237

NEURORADIOLOGY

BT   Diagnosis, radiologic
RT   Nervous system
Neurology
  Encyclopedias, loose-
    leaf   82

NEUROSURGERY

See Nervous system

NEWBORNS

RT   Infants
RT   Pediatrics
Diseases
  Diagnosis 382
  Etiology   382
  Incidence 382
  Pathophysiology 305
  Prognosis 382
  Signs and symptoms 382
  Treatment   305, 382
Drugs (treatment modali-
ty)
  Pharmacology 305
Nursing practice   357
  Nervous system
    History and physical
      examination 258
    Physiology 258
  Nutrition 305
  Obstetrics
    Birth defects   321
  Orthopedics 305
  Physiology 318

NOISE POLLUTION

RT   Air pollution
RT   Ecology
RT   Environmental health

RT   Radiation pollution
Chemical materials, indus-
  trial
  Control   114
  Hazards   114

NOMENCLATURE

RT   Classification systems
RT   Terminology
Anatomy 309
Bacteriology
  Microbiology   251
Biochemistry
  Handbooks   94
Embryology 309
Enzymes
  Classification numbers
    154
  Names, recommended 154
  Names, systemic   154
  Reactions   154
Histology 309
Mental illness   118
Molecular biology
  Handbooks   94
Veterinary medicine
  Anatomy 309
Viruses
  Animals
    Encyclopedias   146

NOMOGRAMS

Body surface area   110,
  253, 418
  Pediatrics   192
Clinical pharmacology
  Drug prescribing   188

NONPROPRIETARY NAMES

See Generic names

NORMAL LABORATORY VALUES

UF   Laboratory values
Tabular data   38, 67, 92,
  104, 105, 110, 111, 145,
  156, 172, 187, 196, 286,
  296, 351, 384, 391, 400,
  415
  Barnes Hospital   253
  Blood 77, 240
  Bone marrow 77
  Encyclopedias, loose-

leaf   81
Nursing practice   239,
312, 313
  Blood   144
Obstetrics   232
Pediatrics   192, 195,
232, 304
  Blood   208
Prenatal care   232
Veterinary medicine
  Cats   113
  Dogs   113

NORMAL VARIATION

Medical genetics   270

NOSE

See Otolaryngology

NOSE DROPS

BT   Drugs
Patient education   280

NOSOCOMIAL INFECTIONS

BT   Communicable diseases
RT   Infection control
Complications   259
Control   259
Diagnosis   259
Epidemiology   259
Etiology   259, 355
Handbooks   354
History   259
Immunology   259
Laboratory science, clini-
cal
  Tabular data   99
Occurrence   259
Pathology   259
Prevention   259, 355
Public health   259
Signs and symptoms   259
Transmission   259
Treatment   259

NUCLEAR MEDICINE

RT   Diagnosis, radiologic
Laboratory science, clini-
cal
  Tabular data   99

NUCLEIC ACIDS

Biochemistry
  Tabular data   94
Microbial composition
  Tabular data   98

NUCLEOTIDES

Biochemistry
  Tabular data   94
Biosynthesis
  Biochemistry   43

NURSES, NUMBER OF

Health personnel, world
  Statistical data   443

NURSING

RT   Journals, nursing
RT   Nursing schools
RT   Nursing practice
RT   Organizations, nursing
Career development
  Job interviewing   317
Dictionaries   145, 246,
296
Directories
  Bibliographies   124
  Certification   303
  Education   303
  Federal health offices
  303
  Licensure   303
  State health offices
  303
Employment possibilities
  Hospitals
    Directories
      Addresses   317
      Beds, number of   317
      Continuing education
      317
      Fringe benefits   317
      Salaries   317
      Telephone numbers
      317
      Working conditions
      317
Encyclopedias   145
Indexes, literature   218,
315
Information sources
  Awards   303

Clearinghouses, health 303
Education 303
Patient information re-
  sources 303
Preventive health 303
Recruitment resources
  303
Scholarships 303
Statistical data
  Distribution 157
  Economic status 157
  Education, nursing 157

NURSING BOARDS

See Boards of nursing

NURSING HOMES

RT Hospitals
Directories
  Addresses 424
  Administrators 424
  Beds, number of 424
  Services 424

NURSING ORGANIZATIONS

See Organizations, nursing

NURSING PRACTICE

RT Nursing
RT Patient education
Abbreviations
  Medical orders
    Latin terms 313
Acid-base disturbances
  Case histories 314
  Laboratory diagnosis
    314
  Nursing care 314
  Signs and symptoms 314
Almanacs 438
Anesthesia 11
Bill of rights, dying per-
  sons
  Texts 438
Bill of rights, patients
  Texts 438
Bill of rights, pregnant
  patients
  Texts 438
Body fluid disturbances
  Case histories 314

Laboratory diagnosis
  314
Nursing care 314
Signs and symptoms 314
Brand names
Dosage and administra-
  tion 313
Formulas 313
Legal status 313
Manufacturers 313
Uses, therapeutic 313
Cardiac rehabilitation
Patient care 62
Cardiovascular drugs
Actions and uses 62
Adverse effects 62
Dosage and administra-
  tion 62
Elimination 62
Indications 62
Metabolism 62
Cardiovascular system
Anatomy 62
Physiology 62
Coronary artery diseases
Diagnosis 62
Pathophysiology 62
Patient assessment 62
Treatment 62
Critical care
Anatomy 100
Cardiac rhythms 295
Crisis management
  Burns 100
  Diabetic emergencies
    100
  Diabetes 100
  Drug overdose 100
  Gastrointestinal
    bleeding 100
  Hepatic failure 100
  Poisoning 100
Critical care units 295
Diseases
  Diagnosis 100
  Pathophysiology 100
  Treatment 100
Drugs (treatment modali-
  ty)
  Adverse effects 295
  Dosage and administra-
    tion 295
  Indications 295
Electrocardiograms
  Interpretations 295
History and physical ex-

amination
 Techniques 295
Holistic approach   100
Infection control   295
Life support
 Techniques 295
Physiology 100
Critical care unit person-
nel
 Job burnout 100
 Job training 100
 Legal aspects 100
 Stress   100
Diagnosis
 Techniques 242
Diagnosis, laboratory
 Abbreviations 239
 Interferences 137, 239,
  312, 313
 Normal ranges 239
 Nursing implications
  239
 Techniques 239
Diseases
 Diagnosis 100, 242, 294
 Epidemiology 277
 Etiology 242, 277
 Incubation periods 144
 Patient advice 242
 Patient care standards
  333
 Signs and symptoms 242,
  277, 333
 Treatment 100, 242,
  277, 294
Drugs
 Actions and uses 137,
  144, 160, 295, 312, 313
 Adverse effects 137,
  160, 295, 312, 313
 Brand names 313
 Cardiovascular drugs 62
 Chemical properties 160
 Classification systems
  312
 Dispensing instructions
  313
 Dosage and administra-
  tion 137, 144, 160,
  295, 312, 313
 Drug interactions 137,
  160, 312, 313
 Excretion 137
 Generic names 160
 Interferences
  Diagnosis, laboratory

  137, 239, 312, 313
 Legal status 313
 Overdose
  Treatment 313
 Patient education 137,
  313
 Pharmacokinetics 137,
  160, 312
 Pharmacology 313
 Physical properties 160
 Pregnancy, use during
  137, 312
 Preparations 144, 160
 Pronunciation 137
 Storage requirements
  312, 313
 Synonyms 160
 Toxicology 160
 Trade names 137, 160
Drugs, nonprescription
 Directions for use 313
 Dosage and administra-
  tion 313
 Formulas 313
Electrolyte disturbances
 Case histories 314
 Laboratory diagnosis
  314
 Nursing care 314
 Signs and symptoms 314
Emergency care
 Assessment 144
 Bites and stings
  Signs and symptoms
  144
  Treatment 144
 Burns
  Assessment, prehospi-
   tal care 144
  Classification systems
   144
  Pathophysiology 144
  Stabilization, emer-
   gency room 144
 Drugs (treatment modali-
  ty) 144
 Food poisoning
  Incubation periods
   144
  Signs and symptoms
   144
 Joint Commission on Ac-
  creditation
  Requirements
   Interpretations 144
   Standards 144

UF-Used For, BT-Broader Term, NT-Narrower Term, RT-Related Term

Life support   144
Nursing role   144
Patient education   144
Poisoning
  Assessment   144
  Life support   144
  Treatment   144
Shock treatment
  Assessment   144
  Complications   144
  Etiology   144
  Pathology   144
  Pathophysiology   144
  Signs and symptoms
    144
  Treatment   144
Toxicology, plants
  Signs and symptoms
    144
  Toxic parts   144
  Treatment   144
Trauma
  Assessment   144
  Diagnosis   144
  Signs and symptoms
    144
  Treatment   144
  Triage   144
  Wound treatment   144
Gynecology
  Anatomy   258
  Physiology   258
  Sexual response   258
Information sources   438
Instruments, surgical
  Atlases   228
Law
  Crimes   241
  Dying declarations   241
  Liabilities   241
  Licensure   241
  Malpractice   241
  Negligence   241
  Professional responsi-
    bilities   241
  Torts   241
  U.S. court system   241
  U.S. governmental struc-
    ture   241
  U.S. jurisprudence   241
  U.S. legislation   241
  Wills   241
  Witnesses   241
Medical records
  Interpretation   167
Nervous system

Anatomy   63
Diseases
  Classification   63
  Diagnostic tests   63
  Examination   63
  Nursing intervention
    63
  Prognosis   63
Embryology   63
Equipment   63
History and physical ex-
  amination   63
Physiology   63
Standards of care   63
Newborn care
  Techniques   357
Normal laboratory values
  Tabular data   312, 313
    Blood   144
Obstetrics
  Abortion   258
  Family structure   258
  Genetic counseling   258
  Infertility   258
  Newborns
    Neurologic assessment
      258
    Physiology   258
  Pregnancy
    Antepartal care   258
    Biophysical aspects
      258
    Childbirth   258
    Complications   258
    Diseases
      Diagnosis   258
      Signs and symptoms
        258
      Treatment   258
    Embryo development
      258
    Embryo physiology   258
    Fetus development   258
    Fetus physiology   258
    Nutrition   258
    Parent education   258
    Postpartum period   258
    Psychosocial aspects
      258
    Risk factors   258
  Sexual counseling   258
Operating room
  Design   11
  Infection control   11
  Nursing service adminis-
    tration   11

Safety 11
Surgical positions of
  patient 11
Ophthalmology
  Anatomy 316
  Diseases
    Nursing care 316
    Signs and symptoms
    316
  Glossaries 316
  Physiology 316
Otolaryngology
  Anatomy 316
  Diseases
    Nursing care 316
    Signs and symptoms
    316
  Glossaries 316
  Physiology 316
Pain
  Differential diagnosis
  63
  Treatment 63
Pediatrics
  Communicable diseases
  296
  Diseases
    Diagnosis 88
    Psychological aspects
    88
    Signs and symptoms 88
    Treatment 88
  Growth and development
  88
  Immunizations
    Schedules 88
  Physiology 88
Pharmacology 160
Procedures 167, 294
Sexuality
  Abortion 214
  Assessment 214
  Contraception 214
  Disease states (during)
  214
  Drug effects 214
  Dysfunction
    Etiology 214
    Treatment 214
  Infertility 214
  Life cycle 214
  Pregnancy 214
  Sexual assault 214
  Sexually transmitted
  diseases 214
Tabular data

Weights and measures
  313
Travel
  Recommendations 313
  Requirements 313
Treatment, surgical 277
  Anesthesia 11
  Patient education 11
  Techniques 11
  Wound healing 11

NURSING SCHOOLS

BT   University programs
RT   Education, nursing
RT   Nursing
  Addresses 341
  Chairpersons 341
  Directors 303
  Expenses 341
  Faculty, number of 341
  Information sources 303
  Programs offered 341
  Ratings 176, 177
  Statistical data 303
  Students, number of 341
  Telephone numbers 341
  University community 341

NURSING SERVICE ADMINISTRA-
TION

  Operating room
    Nursing care 11

NUTRITION

NT   Parenteral nutrition
RT   Caffeine content
RT   Catabolism
RT   Cholesterol content
RT   Dietetics, clinical
RT   Diets, modified
RT   Foods
RT   Lipids
RT   Malnutrition
RT   Metabolism
RT   Minerals
RT   Nutritional content
RT   Nutritional deficien-
       cies
RT   Purines
RT   Recommended dietary al-
       lowances
RT   Vitamins
  Bacteriology 39

Biochemistry   403
Biology
  Tabular data   48
CRC handbooks
  Indexes   93
Encyclopedias, loose-leaf
  81
Family practice   281
Food supply
  Toxicology
    Chemical additives
      293
Gastrointestinal system
  169
  Pediatrics   335
Laboratory animal sciences
  Handbooks   97
Minerals
  Metabolism   293
  Requirements   293
Newborns   305
Pathophysiology   331
Pediatrics   108, 192, 304,
  339
  Tabular data   195
Pregnancy
  Nursing practice   258
Prevention
  Diseases   293
Public health   259
Requirements
  Adolescence   293
  Aged   293
  Environmental stress
    293
  Exercise stress   293
  Infancy   293
  Pregnancy   293
  Work stress   293
Statistical data   390
Tabular data
  Handbooks   170
Treatment, surgical
  Abdomen   4
  Handbooks   110
Vitamins
  Metabolism   293
  Requirements   293
  Toxicology   293

NUTRITIONAL CONTENT

RT   Nutrition
  Foods
    Amino acids   54, 245
    Cholesterol   54, 187,
      245
    Fatty acids   187, 245
    Fluoride   54
    Folacin   187
    Inorganic constituents 245
    Iodine   245
    Minerals   54
    Organic acids   245
    Phytic acid   245
    Proximate composition   54,
      245
    Tabular data   170
    Vitamins   54, 245
    Zinc   54, 187

NUTRITIONAL DEFICIENCIES

UF   Deficiencies, nutritional
RT   Malnutrition
  Minerals   293, 296
  Tropical medicine
    Control   215
    Diagnosis   215
    Distribution   215
    Etiology   215
    History   215
    Pathogenesis   215
    Pathophysiology   215
    Prevention   215
    Prognosis   215
    Signs and symptoms   215
    Treatment   215
  Vitamins   293, 296, 350
    Signs and symptoms   175

OBESITY

UF   Overweight
  Anesthesia
    Pathophysiology   28
  Differential diagnosis   244
  Endocrine system   405
  Gynecology   76
  Malnutrition   293

OBSTETRICS

RT   Abortion
RT   Antepartal care
RT   Childbirth
RT   Fetus
RT   Gynecology
RT   Postpartum period
RT   Pregnancy
RT   Puerperium
RT   Reproduction

Anatomy 441
Contraception 441
Cytopathology 310
Diseases
  Endocrine system 310,
  441
  Pathology 310
  Signs and symptoms
  310
  Treatment 441
Embryology 310
Endocrine system 441
Fetus
  Monitoring 441
  Prenatal care 191, 305,
  441
Genetics 318
Histology 310
History 318
Home birth 191
Newborns
  Birth defects 321
Normal laboratory values
232
Nursing practice
  Abortion 258
  Family structure 258
  Genetic counseling 258
  Infertility 258
  Pregnancy 258
Pathology
  Abortion 310
Physiology 441
Pregnancy
  Childbirth 191
  Complications 191, 310,
  441
  Diagnosis 191
  Emotional aspects 191
  Home delivery 191
  Pathology 310
  Physiology 441
Puerperium 441
Sterilization
  Indications 191
  Techniques 191
Treatment, surgical
  Analgesia 321
  Anatomy 321
  Anesthesia 321
  Childbirth 321
  Postoperative care 321
  Postoperative complica-
  tions 321
  Prenatal care 321
  Preoperative care 321

Techniques 321
Urology
  Diseases
    Diagnosis 185
    Treatment 185

OCCUPANCY, PERCENTAGE

  Hospitals
    Statistical data 184,
    212

OCCUPATIONAL DISEASES

  RT Occupational health
  Biological hazards
    Adverse effects 319
    Prevention 319
    Routes of entry 319
  Chemical hazards 114
    Adverse effects 319
    Diagnostic tests 319
    Permissible exposure
    limits 319
    Personnel protective
    measures 319
    Routes of entry 319
  Pesticides
    Adverse effects 319
    Laboratory diagnosis
    319
    Permissible exposure
    limits 319
    Treatment 319
  Physical hazards
    Adverse effects 319
    Routes of entry 319
  Signs and symptoms
    Indexes 220

OCCUPATIONAL HEALTH

  RT Chemical hazards
  RT Environmental health
  RT Industrial hazards
  RT Occupational diseases
  RT Ventilation procedures
  Disability, physical 237
  U.S. government documents
    Indexes 282
  Public health
    Regulations 259

OCCUPATIONAL MEDICINE

  Encyclopedias, loose-leaf

81

OCCUPATIONAL THERAPY

  RT   Physical therapy
  RT   Rehabilitation
   Abbreviations   3
   Allied health sciences
      Indexes, literature   315
   Diseases
      Rheumatology   84
   Undergraduate schools
      Ratings   177

OCULAR MANIFESTATIONS

  RT   Ophthalmology
   Diseases   323
      Pediatrics   336
   Systemic diseases   171,
   323

OFFICE DESIGN

   Practice management
      Family medicine   406

OFFICIALS

  RT   Administrators
  RT   Chairpersons
  RT   Contact persons
  RT   Deans
  RT   Directors
  RT   Executives
   American College of Physi-
   cians   45
   American College of Sur-
   geons   16
   American Dental Associa-
   tion   17
   American Hospital Associa-
   tion   184
   American Medical Associa-
   tion   14
   American Psychiatry Associa-
   tion   44
   American specialty boards
   126
   Association of American
   Medical Colleges   2
   Foundations   163
   Governmental agencies
   299, 423
   Medical schools   2, 275
   Organizations   147

   Organizations, dental,
   state   17
   Research institutes, foreign   445
   Research programs, biomedical sciences   376
   Research programs, dental
   376
   Research programs, medical
   376
   Research programs, pharmacology   376
   Research programs, veterinary medicine   376

OLD AGE

   See Aged

OLIGONUCLEOTIDES

   Biochemistry
      Tabular data   94

ONCOLOGY

   See Cancer

OPERATING ROOM

  RT   Instruments, surgical
  RT   Treatment, surgical
   Dental care
      Hospitals   210
   Nursing care
      Design   11
      Infection control   11
      Nursing service adminis-
      tration   11
      Safety   11
      Surgical positions of
      patient   11

OPHTHALMOLOGY

  UF   Eyes
  NT   Neuro-ophthalmology
  RT   Ocular manifestations
  RT   Visual systems
   Abbreviations   323
   Anatomy   171, 323
   Biochemistry   323
   Diagnostic techniques   171
   Diseases
      Classification systems
      171

Diagnosis   322, 323
Etiology   171
Pathology   171
Prognosis   171
Signs and symptoms   171, 323
Treatment   171, 323
Treatment, surgical
    Indications   322
    Techniques   322
Embryology   323
Glossaries   323
Growth and development 171
History and physical examination   171, 323
Nursing practice
    Anatomy   316
    Diseases
        Nursing care   316
        Signs and symptoms 316
        Glossaries   316
        Physiology   316
Pediatrics
    Diseases
        Diagnosis   336
        Drugs (treatment modality)
            Dosage and administration   336
        Signs and symptoms 336
        Treatment   336
Physiology   323
Preventive medicine   171
Treatment, surgical
    Anesthesia   322
    Diagnosis   322
    Informed consent   322
    Instrumentation   322
    Patient education   322
    Postoperative care   322
    Preoperative antibiotics 322
    Preoperative care   322
    Preoperative cultures 322
    Sutures   322
    Techniques   322

ORAL DISEASES

RT   Dentistry
RT   Mouth
Drugs (treatment modality)

Actions and uses   5
Adverse effects   5
Chemical descriptions   5
Distributors   5
Trade names   5
Warnings   5
Prevention   5
Treatment, surgical
    Anesthesia   409
    Techniques   409

ORAL MANIFESTATIONS

RT   Dentistry
RT   Mouth
Diseases, metabolic   410
Systemic diseases   410
    Diagnosis   399
    Epidemiology   399
    Etiology   399
    Illustrations   399
    Pathogenesis   399
    Prognosis   399
    Treatment   399

ORDERING INFORMATION

RT   Catalogs
Audiovisual materials   300
Books   265
Journals   265, 420
Organizations
    Publications   385
Proceedings, published 127, 221
Reagents   307
U.S. government documents 282

ORGAN DONATIONS

Death and dying   389
Directories   381

ORGAN PRESERVATION

Transplantation   360

ORGANIC ACID COMPOSITION

Foods   245

ORGANIC COMPOUNDS

RT   Inorganic compounds
Tabular data   95

UF-Used For, BT-Broader Term, NT-Narrower Term, RT-Related Term

ORGANIZATIONAL CHARTS

    Governmental agencies   423

ORGANIZATIONS

   UF Associations
   NT Organizations, dental
   NT Organizations, dental,
      state
   NT Organizations, medical
   NT Organizations, nursing
   NT Organizations, pharma-
      cology
   NT Organizations, veteri-
      nary medicine
   Directories   381
     Activities   446
     Financial data   446
     Founding dates   446
     Languages   446
     Meeting dates   446
     Members, number of   446
     Patient education
       Addresses   90
     Publications   446
     Staff, number of   446

ORGANIZATIONS, DENTAL

   BT Organizations
   NT Canadian Dental Associ-
      ation
   NT Council on Dental Ther-
      apeutics
   RT Dentistry
   Activities   151
   Addresses   17, 151
   Founding dates   151
   Members, number of   151
   Staff, number of   151
   Telephone numbers   17, 151

ORGANIZATIONS, DENTAL, STATE

   BT Organizations
   Addresses   17

ORGANIZATIONS, MEDICAL

   UF Health organizations
   BT Organizations
   NT American Board of Sur-
      gery
   NT American College of
      Physicians

   NT American College of
      Surgeons
   NT American Hospital Asso-
      ciation
   NT American Medical Asso-
      ciation
   NT American Psychiatry As-
      sociation
   NT American Public health
      Association
   NT American specialty
      boards
   NT Association of American
      Medical Colleges
   NT Association of Cancer
      Centers
   NT Voluntary health organ-
      izations
   Abbreviations   3, 119
   Acronyms   147
   Activities   147, 151, 198
   Addresses   58, 147, 151,
    198, 261
   Awards   198
   Descriptions   261
   Directors   198, 261
   Founding dates   147, 151,
    198
   Journals   261
   Meeting dates   147, 198
   Meeting locations   147,
    198
   Members, number of   147,
    151, 198, 261
   Membership fees   198
   Officials   147, 184
   Publications   147, 198,
    261
     Ordering information
     385
   Purposes   198
   Staff, number of 151
   Telephone numbers   58,
    147, 151, 184, 198, 261

ORGANIZATIONS, NURSING

   UF Nursing organizations
   BT Organizations
   RT Nursing
   Directories   303
     Activities   151, 157
     Addresses   151, 157,
     246, 296
     Founding dates   151
     Members, number of   151

Staff, number of   151
Telephone numbers   151

ORGANIZATIONS, PHARMACOLOGY

UF   Pharmacology organiza-
     tions
BT   Organizations
Activities   151
Addresses   136, 151
Contact persons   136
Founding dates   151
Members, number of   151
Staff, numbers of   151
Telephone numbers   136,
151

ORGANIZATIONS, SCIENTIFIC

UF   Scientific organiza-
     tions
BT   Organizations
Acronyms   147
Activities   147
Addresses   147
Founding dates   147
Meeting dates   147
Meeting locations   147
Members, number of 147
Officials   147
Publications   147
Telephone numbers   147

ORIGIN OF LIFE

Biochemistry   43

ORIGINAL ARTICLES

RT   History
RT   Medical firsts
Bibliographies
  Diagnostic techniques
  152
  Diseases   71, 152, 217
    Metabolism   368
    Physician biographies
    71
  Strains   152
  Syndromes   121, 217, 368
  Treatment, surgical
    Techniques   152

ORTHOPEDICS

RT   Birth fractures

RT   Bones
RT   Dislocations
RT   Fracture-dislocations
RT   Fractures
RT   Muscles
RT   Synovial joints
Amputations
  Dictionaries   326
  Treatment, surgical
    Techniques   56
Arthrodesis
  Treatment, surgical
    Techniques   56
Arthroplasty
  Treatment, surgical
    Techniques   56
Atlases
  Birth fractures
    Diagnosis   115
    Mechanism of action
    115
    Treatment   115
  Dislocations
    Diagnosis   115
    Mechanism of injury
    115
    Treatment   115
  Fracture-dislocations
    Diagnosis   115
    Mechanism of injury
    115
    Treatment   115
  Fractures
    Diagnosis   115
    Mechanism of injury
    115
    Treatment   115
  Subluxations
    Diagnosis   115
    Mechanism of injury
    115
    Treatment   115
Dictionaries   326
  Abbreviations   254
  Amputation   326
  Anatomy   254
  Diagnostic techniques
  254
  Diseases   254
    Diagnosis   326
    Etiology   326
    Pathology   326
    Signs and symptoms
    326
    Treatment   326
  Fractures   254

UF-Used For, BT-Broader Term, NT-Narrower Term, RT-Related Term

Physical medicine 254
Positions, anatomical
  254
Skin grafting 326
Tests 254
Treatment 254
Diseases
  Anatomy 327
  Diagnosis, radiologic
    327
  Etiology 327
  Pathogenesis 327
  Prognosis 327
  Treatment 327
  Treatment, surgical
    Techniques 56
Dislocations
  Classification systems
    165
  Complications 165
  Diagnosis 115, 165
  Dictionaries 254
  Historical backgrounds
    165
  Mechanism of injury 115
  Pathological anatomy
    165
  Treatment 115, 165
  Treatment, surgical
    Techniques 56
Embryology 327
Fractures
  Anatomy 327
  Atlases 115
  Classification systems
    165
  Complications 165
  Diagnosis 115, 165
  Diagnosis, radiologic
    327
  Etiology 327
  Historical background
    165
  Mechanism of injury 115
  Pathogenesis 327
  Pathological anatomy
    165
  Prognosis 327
  Treatment 115, 165, 327
  Treatment, surgical
    Techniques 56
Histology 327
Injuries
  Classification systems
    165
  Complications 165

Diagnosis 165
Historical background
  165
Pathological anatomy
  165
Treatment 165
Newborns 305
Pediatrics
  Diseases
    Diagnosis 337
    Etiology 337
    Pathology 337
    Signs and symptoms
      337
    Treatment 337
  Dislocations
    Mechanism of injury
      337
    Pathologic anatomy
      337
    Treatment 337
  Fractures
    Mechanism of injury
      337
    Pathologic anatomy
      337
    Treatment 337
    Treatment, surgical
      Techniques 337
  Physiology 327

OTOLARYNGOLOGY

UF   Ear
UF   Nose
UF   Throat
RT   Head
RT   Neck
Anatomy 328, 411
Biochemistry 328
Diseases
  Diagnosis 328, 411
  Etiology 328
  Pathology 328
  Signs and symptoms 328
  Treatment 328, 411
Embryology 328
Histology 328
History and physical exam-
  ination 328, 411
Microbiology 328
Nursing practice
  Anatomy 316
  Diseases
    Nursing care 316
    Signs and symptoms

316
  Glossaries 316
  Physiology 316
Pathology 328
Physiology 328, 411
Plastic surgery
  Techniques 328
Reconstructive surgery
  Techniques 328

OUTPATIENT SURGERY

  BT Treatment, surgical
  RT Ambulatory medicine
  Anesthesia 233

OUTPATIENT VISITS

  RT Ambulatory medicine
  Hospitals
    Statistical data 212

OVER THE COUNTER DRUGS

  See Drugs, nonprescription

OVERDOSAGE

  RT Adverse effects
  RT Poisoning
  Drugs 158
    Nursing practice 100, 313
  Drugs, nonprescription
    Signs and symptoms 349
    Treatment 349

OVERWEIGHT

  See Obesity

PACKAGING

  RT Dosage and administration
  Cultures
    Procedures 65
    Regulations 65
  Drugs 18, 138, 158, 371, 426
    Catalogs 19, 136
  Drugs, new 138

PAIN

  Anesthesia 27, 233

Differential diagnosis 244
Nervous system
  Physiology 306
  Treatment 306
Nursing practice
  Differential diagnosis 63
  Treatment 63

PAIN CENTERS

  Directories 203

PALLOR

  Differential diagnosis 244

PAMPHLETS

  Bibliography, annotated
    Patient education 90

PANCREAS

  RT Digestion
  RT Endocrine system
  Diseases
    Treatment, surgical
      Techniques 393

PARASITOLOGY

  RT Animal hosts
  RT Helminths
  RT Protozoa
  Animals
    Encyclopedias 146
  Arthropods
    Biology 83
    Classification systems 83
    Diagnosis, immunologic 83
    Diseases
      Diagnosis 83
      Epidemiology 83
      Pathogenesis 83
      Pathology 83
      Prevention 83
      Prognosis 83
      Signs and symptoms 83
      Treatment 83
    Entomologic methods 83
    History 83

  Illustrations 83
  Life cycles 83
  Morphology 83
  Specimen examination
   techniques 83
Biology
  Tabular data 48
Diagnosis, laboratory
  Interpretations of tests
   179
  Laboratory techniques
   179
Diseases
  Diagnosis 168
  Treatment 168
Helminths
  Biology 83
  Classification systems
   83
  Diagnosis, immunologic
   83
  Diseases
   Diagnosis 83
   Epidemiology 83
   Pathogenesis 83
   Pathology 83
   Prevention 83
   Prognosis 83
   Signs and symptoms 83
   Treatment 83
  Entomologic methods 83
  History 83
  Illustrations 83
  Life cycles 83
  Morphology 83
  Specimen examination
   techniques 83
Laboratory science, clini-
 cal
  Tabular data
   Handbooks 99
Microbiology
  Assays 251
  Characterization 251
  Culture and isolation
   251
  Examination 251
  Identifications 251
  Interpretations 251
  Serodiagnosis 251
  Tests 251
Protozoa
  Biology 83
  Classification systems
   83
  Diagnosis, immunologic
   83
  Diseases
   Diagnosis 83
   Epidemiology 83
   Pathogenesis 83
   Pathology 83
   Prevention 83
   Prognosis 83
   Signs and symptoms 83
   Treatment 83
  Entomologic methods 83
  History 83
  Illustrations 83
  Life cycles 83
  Morphology 83
  Specimen examination
   techniques 83

PARENTERAL NUTRITION

  BT Nutrition
  Clinical pharmacology
   Handbooks 188
  Pediatrics
   Treatment, surgical 397

PATENT DEPOSITORY LIBRARIES

  Directories
   Addresses 129
   Telephone numbers 129

PATHOGENESIS

  RT Etiology
  RT Pathologic microorga-
       nisms
  RT Pathology
  Diseases 329
   Ambulatory medicine 358
   Birth defects 49
   Cancer 60
   Communicable diseases
    223, 355
    Pediatrics 224
    Treatment, surgical
     395
    Tropical medicine 215
   Dermatology 26, 116
   Electrolyte disturbances
    372
   Fractures 327
   Gastrointestinal system
    75
   Genetics 287
   Genitourinary system 172

Hematology   77, 207,
  240
Kidney   236, 372
Nervous system   306
Orthopedics   327
Parasitology
  Arthropods 83
  Helminths 83
  Protozoa 83
Pediatrics
  Gastrointestinal sys-
    tem 335
Respiratory system   117,
  413
Rheumatology 31
Tropical medicine   215
Veterinary medicine
  Cattle 432
  Horses 432
  Pigs 432
  Sheep 432

PATHOGENIC MICROORGANISMS

RT Pathogenesis
 Microbiology
  Cultivation 35
  Diagnosis
    Serologic procedures
      35
  Identification
    Atlases 35
    Procedures 35

PATHOLOGY

NT Cytopathology
NT Histopathology
NT Immunopathology
RT Etiology
RT Forensic pathologists
RT Pathogenesis
RT Pathology, surgical
RT Pathophysiology
 Body fluids 330
 Cell injury 329, 330
 Classification systems
  Diseases 398
  Etiology 398
  Morphology 398
  Occupations 398
  Physiology 398
  Services 347
  Techniques 347, 398
  Topography 398
 Diseases   67, 73, 288,

329, 330, 415
Abortion 310
Bile ducts 133
Cancer 7, 60, 61
Communicable diseases
  223, 259
  Pediatrics 224
Dermatology 116
Dictionaries 217
Emergency care 142
Encyclopedias, loose-
  leaf 81
Endocrine system 405
Family medicine 406
Food poisoning 259
Gallbladder 133
Gastrointestinal system
  75, 169
Genetics 329
Gynecology 191, 310,
  311
Immunology 329
Inflammation 329, 330
Liver 132, 133
Nervous system 408
  Encyclopedias, loose-
    leaf 82
Nosocomial infections
  259
Obstetrics 310
Ophthalmology 171
Orthopedics 165, 326,
  337
Otolaryngology 328
Parasitology
  Arthropods 83
  Helminths 83
  Protozoa 83
Pediatrics 304, 339
  Orthopedics 337
Poisoning (of humans)
  Animals, marine 352
Pregnancy, abnormal 310
Respiratory system 117,
  365
Rheumatology 31, 414
Sexually transmitted
  diseases 259
Snakebites
  Tropical medicine 215
Veterinary medicine 433
  Cattle 432
  Horses 432
  Pigs 432
  Sheep 432
Physiology

UF–Used For, BT–Broader Term, NT–Narrower Term, RT–Related Term

Allergy 388
Cardiorenal system 388
Communicable diseases
 388
Endocrine system 388
Gastrointestinal system
 388
Hematology 388
Metabolism 388
Respiratory system 388
Rheumatology 388
Toxicology 388
Syndromes 121, 217

PATHOLOGY, SURGICAL

RT Pathology
RT Treatment, surgical
Diseases
  Gross characteristics
    Atlases 8
  Histology
    Atlases 8
Specimen handling tech-
 niques 8

PATHOPHYSIOLOGY

NT Physiology
RT Pathology
Acid-base disturbances
 236
Anesthesia 28
Blood 331
Burns
  Emergency care
    Nursing practice 144
Cell biology 331
Connective tissue 331
Diseases 38, 331, 360,
 388
  Anesthesia 28
  Biochemistry 403
  Blood vessels 205
  Cardiovascular system
   62, 331, 417
  Communicable diseases
    Tropical medicine 215
  Critical care
    Nursing practice 100
  Dermatology 26, 116,
   331
  Drugs, nonprescription
    Handbooks 190
  Electrolyte disturbances
   74, 236, 392

Emergency care 142, 143
  Anesthesia 28
  Pediatrics 412
Encyclopedias 196
Encyclopedias, loose-
 leaf 81
Endocrine system 153,
 331
Fluid disturbances 74,
 236
Gastrointestinal system
 75, 168, 169, 331
Genetics 287, 331
Heart 205, 206
Hypertension 331
Immunology 331
Kidney 236, 331, 392
Liver 331
Metabolism 331
Nervous system 306, 331
Newborns 305
Nutrition 331
  Tropical medicine 215
Respiratory system 331
Rheumatology 31
Small animals
  Veterinary medicine
   113
Thorax 417
Tropical medicine
  Nutritional deficien-
   cies 215
  Poisoning (of humans)
    Fish 215
    Plants 215

PATIENT CARE STANDARDS

Diseases
  Nursing practice 333

PATIENT EDUCATION

UF Consumer health
RT Nursing practice
Accidents
  First aid 21
Adolescence 21
Aged 21
Anatomy 21
Bibliography, annotated
  Books 90
  Pamphlets 90
Directories
  Addresses
    Audiovisual producers

90
  Governmental agencies
  90
  Insurance companies
  90
  Organizations 90
  Voluntary health or-
  ganizations 90
Childbirth 21
Contraception 21
Death and dying 21
Diseases
  Activity restrictions
  227
  Descriptions 227
  Diagnosis 21
  Diet therapy 227
  Family practice 281
  Medication instructions
  227
  Medication precautions
  227
  Nursing practice 242
  Prognosis 21
  Signs and symptoms 21
  Treatment 21
  Warning signs of compli-
  cations 227
Drugs 137, 188, 313
  Actions and uses 280,
  427
  Adverse effects 21,
  280, 427
  Brand names 427
  Dosage and administra-
  tion 21, 280
  Generic names 21
  Pronunciations 427
  Storage recommendations
  280
  Trade names 21
  Warnings 280
    Breast feeding 427
    Cross-sensitivity 427
    Drug interactions 427
    Pregnancy 427
Drugs, nonprescription
90, 190
Ear drops
  Drugs 280
Emergency care
  First aid 21
  Nursing practice 144
Eye drops
  Drugs 280
Eye ointments

Drugs 280
Family medicine 406
Health care system 21
Infertility 21
Information sources 90,
145
Nose drops
  Drugs 280
Ophthalmology
  Treatment, surgical 322
Pregnancy 21
Rectal suppositories
  Drugs 280
Self-treatment 349
Sexuality 21
Treatment, surgical
  Nursing care 11
U.S. government documents
  Ordering information
  282

PATIENT RIGHTS

UF Rights of patients
RT Bill of rights, dying
    persons
RT Bill of rights, pa-
    tients
RT Bill of rights, preg-
    nant patients
RT Informed consent
RT Law
  Death and dying 389
  Texts (Bill of Rights) 6,
  120

PEDIATRICS

UF Children, care of
RT Adolescence
RT Infants
RT Newborns
RT Runaway youth centers
  Accidents
    Treatment 108, 109
  Almanacs 439
  Ambulatory care 108
  Anesthesia 233
    Agent selection 29
    Blood replacement 29
    Complications 29
    Dentistry 29
    Fluid therapy 29
    Intensive care 29
    Legal aspects 29
    Monitoring 29

Mortality 29
Techniques 29
Treatment, surgical 29
Birth defects
  Classification systems
    339
  Screening 339
Bites and stings
  Signs and symptoms 304
  Treatment 109, 304
Burns
  Treatment 109
Communicable diseases
  Communicability periods
    296
  Complications 224, 296
  Control 296
  Diagnosis 224, 373
  Differential diagnosis
    224
  Epidemiology 224
  Etiology 224, 373
  Immunizations 224
  Incubation periods 296
  Nursing practice 296
  Pathogenesis 224
  Pathology 224
  Prognosis 224
  Signs and symptoms 224,
    296
  Sources 296
  Transmission 296
  Treatment 224, 296, 373
Death and dying
  Medicolegal investiga-
    tions 292
Dental care
  Hospitals 210
Diagnosis
  Techniques 195
Directories
  Services
    Addresses 297
    Contact persons 297
    Telephone numbers 297
Diseases
  Complications 339
  Diagnosis 108, 192,
    304, 339, 439
  Diagnosis, laboratory
    Indications 232
    Interferences 232
    Interpretations 232
  Diagnosis, radiologic
    338
  Differential diagnosis

108, 192
  Epidemiology 339
  Etiology 304, 339
  Ocular manifestations
    336
  Pathology 304, 339
  Prevention 304, 339
  Prognosis 108, 192,
    304, 339
  Signs and symptoms 108,
    192, 304, 339, 439
  Techniques 195, 412
  Treatment 108, 109,
    192, 304, 339
  Treatment, surgical 397
Drugs
  Adverse effects 195
  Dosage and administra-
    tion 195, 304
  Generic names 195
  Indications 195
  Trade names 195
Emergency care
  Assessment, prehospital
    143
  Differential diagnosis
    412
  Drugs (treatment modali-
    ty)
    Adverse effects 412
    Dosage and administra-
      tion 412
    Routes of administra-
      tion 412
    Warnings 412
  Facility administration
    412
  Instructions to parents
    252
  Pathophysiology 143,
    412
  Resuscitation
    Techniques 412
  Signs and symptoms 143,
    192, 252, 412
  Stabilization, emer-
    gency room 143
  Techniques
    Illustrations 412
  Treatment 108, 143,
    192, 252, 412
Ethics 339
Family medicine 406
Food values
  Tabular data 304
Gastrointestinal system

Diagnosis
  Techniques   335
Diseases
  Diagnosis   335
  Nutritional support
    335
  Pathogenesis   335
  Signs and symptoms
    335
  Treatment   335
Growth and development
  108, 192, 195, 304, 339,
  439
Gynecology   106, 304
  Anatomy   186
  Diseases
    Signs and symptoms
      186
    Treatment   186
  Embryology   186
  History and physical ex-
    amination   186
  Physiology   186
  Sexuality   186
Hematology
  Blood storage   208
  Blood transfusions   208
  Cell biology   208
  Coagulation factors   208
  Diseases
    Prognosis   208
    Treatment   208
  Genetics   208
  Molecular biology   208
  Normal laboratory values
    208
  Signs and symptoms   208
History and physical exam-
  ination   108, 192, 248
Immunizations
  Communicable diseases
    373
  Schedules   108
  Vaccines   108
  Warnings   108
Mental health services
  Addresses   297
  Contact persons   297
  Telephone numbers   297
Nomograms
  Body surface area   192
Normal laboratory values
  Tabular data   192, 195,
    232, 304
  Blood   208
Nursing practice

Diseases
  Diagnosis   88
  Psychological aspects
    88
  Signs and symptoms   88
  Treatment   88
Growth and development
  88
Immunizations
  Schedules   88
Physiology   88
Nutrition   108, 192, 195,
  304, 339
Ophthalmology
  Diagnosis
    Techniques   336
  Diseases
    Diagnosis   336
    Drugs (treatment mo-
      dality)
      Dosage and adminis-
        tration   336
    Signs and symptoms
      336
    Treatment   336
Orthopedics
  Diseases
    Diagnosis   337
    Etiology   337
    Pathology   337
    Signs and symptoms
      337
    Treatment   337
  Dislocations
    Mechanisms of injury
      337
    Pathologic anatomy
      337
    Treatment   337
  Fractures
    Mechanisms of injury
      337
    Pathologic anatomy
      337
    Treatment   337
  Treatment, surgical
    Techniques   337
Poisoning   439
  Etiology   195
  Signs and symptoms   192,
    195, 304
  Treatment   108, 109,
    192, 195, 304
Psychological tests   195
Speech disorders
  Diagnosis   411

UF–Used For, BT–Broader Term, NT–Narrower Term, RT–Related Term

Tabular data
  Blood pressure 195
  Conversion formulas 195
  Growth tables 195
  Normal laboratory values
    195
  Nutrition 195
Toxicology 439
Treatment facilities
  Addresses 297
  Contact persons 297
  Telephone numbers 297
Treatment, surgical
  Body fluid disturbances
    397
  Electrolyte disturbances
    397
  Emotional aspects 397
  History and physical ex-
    amination 397
  Infections, postopera-
    tive 397
  Parenteral nutrition
    397
  Postoperative care 397
  Preoperative care 397
  Respiratory system 397
  Techniques 397

PEPTIDES

  RT   Amino acids
  RT   Polypeptides
  RT   Proteins
  Biochemistry
    Tabular data 94

PERFUMES

  RT   Commercial products,
        chemicals
  RT   Household products
  Prices (retail & whole-
    sale)
    Catalogs
      Drug store merchandise
        136

PERIODICAL LITERATURE INDEXES

  See Indexes, literature

PERIODICALS

  See Journals

PERSONALITY DEVELOPMENT

  BT   Growth and development
  Psychiatry 291

PERSONNEL, HEALTH, WORLD

  See Health personnel, world

PESTICIDES

  BT   Chemicals
  RT   Insecticides
  Chemical names
    Synonyms 342
  Occupational diseases
    Adverse effects 319
    Laboratory diagnosis
      319
    Permissible exposure
      limits 319
    Treatment 319
  Pharmacological names
    Synonyms 342
  Toxicology
    Pharmacology 175
    Signs and symptoms 175
    Treatment 175
  Trade names
    Synonyms 342

pH

  Durgs, injectable 194

PHAGOCYTIC CELLS

  Immunology 37

PHARMACEUTICAL COMPANIES

  See Manufacturers, drugs

PHARMACEUTICAL INGREDIENTS

  RT   Drugs
  Assays 426
  Formulas 426
  Identification 426
  Packaging 426
  Physical characteristics
    426
  Storage 426

PHARMACEUTICAL PRACTICE

RT   Drugs
 Chemistry 371
 Drug interactions   371
 Economics 371
 Legislation 371
 Manufacturers, drugs
   Packaging 371
   Preformulations 371
   Sterilization 371
 Patient care 371
 Poison control 371
 Radioisotopes 371

PHARMACISTS

RT   Pharmacology
 Directories
   Activities, research
   343
   Addresses 343
   Birth dates 343
   Career backgrounds 343
   Educational backgrounds
   343
   Professional memberships
   343
   Publications 343
   Telephone numbers   343

PHARMACOKINETICS

UF   Absorption and fate
     (drugs)
UF   Elimination
RT   Actions and uses
RT   Excretion
 Drugs 15, 20, 138, 158,
   175, 428
   Handbooks 188
   Nursing practice 137,
   160
 Drugs, European 257
 Drugs, new 138
 Drugs (treatment modality)
   Diseases 30
     Allergy 12
     Nursing practice 160,
     312
     Rheumatology 31, 414
 Heavy metals
   Toxicology 175
 Vitamins 175

PHARMACOLOGICAL NAMES

UF   Names, pharmacological

RT   Generic names
RT   Trade names
 Chemical compounds
   Synonyms 342
 Drugs
   Synonyms 342
 Pesticides
   Synonyms 342

PHARMACOLOGY

NT   Clinical pharmacology
RT   Drugs
RT   Pharmacists
 Abbreviations 9
 Acronyms 9
 Air pollutants
   Toxicology 175
 Directories
   Bibliographies 124
   Research programs 376
 Encyclopedias, loose-leaf
   81
 Initialisms 9

PHARMACOLOGY ORGANIZATIONS

See Organizations, pharmacology

PHARMACOPEIAL CONVENTION,
U.S.

See U.S. Pharmacopeial Convention

PHARMACY BOARDS, STATE

See Boards of pharmacy,
state

PHARMACY SCHOOLS

UF   Education, pharmacology
BT   University programs
 Directories
   Addresses 341
   Chairpersons 341
   Expenses 341
   Faculty, number of 341
   Programs 341
   Ratings 176
   Students, number of 341
   Telephone numbers 341
   University community
   341

UF-Used For, BT-Broader Term, NT-Narrower Term, RT-Related Term

PHRASES, MEDICAL

   Keyword indexes   271

PHYSICAL EXAMINATION

  See History and physical
  examination

PHYSICAL THERAPY

  RT   Occupational therapy
  RT   Rehabilitation
  Abbreviations   3
  Disability, physical   237
  Indexes, literature   315
  Rheumatology 84
  Undergraduate schools
    Ratings   177

PHYSICIANS

  NT   Coroners
  NT   Forensic pathologists
  NT   Physicians, women
  NT   Physicians, United
    Kingdom
  RT   American College of
    Physicians
  RT   American College of
    Surgeons
  RT   American Medical Asso-
    ciation
  RT   American Psychiatry As-
    sociation
  RT   American specialty
    boards
  RT   Specialties
  Directories
    Addresses 22, 126, 424
    American specialty board
     certification   22, 126,
     424
    Birth dates   126, 424
    Birth places   126
    Educational backgrounds
     22, 126, 424
    Practice types   22
    Professional memberships
     126, 424
    Provisional certifica-
     tions   126
    Telephone numbers   126
    Year of licensure   22
  History
    Biographies   47, 71, 234

    Statistical data   443
    Fees   363
    Geographic distribution
     346
    Incomes, net   363
    Personal characteristics
     346
    Professional activities
     346
    Professional expenses
     363
    Specialties   346
    Work patterns   363

PHYSICIANS, UNITED KINGDOM

  BT   Physicians
  Directories
    Addresses   268, 274
    Dates of registration
     274
    Professional degrees
     268
    Professional memberships
     268
    Registration numbers
     274
    Telephone numbers   268

PHYSICIANS, WOMEN

  BT   Physicians
  Directories
    Addresses   130
    Educational backgrounds
     130
    Professional backgrounds
     130
    Specialties   130

PHYSICS

  CRC handbooks
    Indexes   93
    Glossaries   95
    Tabular data   95

PHYSIOLOGY

  NT   Neurophysiology
  NT   Pathophysiology
  RT   Anatomy
  Abbreviations   9, 378
  Acronyms   9
  Adrenals   57
  Aged   72, 272

Allergic response   73
Allergy   12
Atlases   70
Bacteriology   39
Body fluid disturbances
  74
Body fluids   272
  Blood   40
  Lymph   40
  Urine excretion   40
Body parts   181, 402, 407
Body systems   181, 402,
  407
Cardiovascular system
  Nursing practice   62
Cells   272, 378
Childbirth   441
Circulation   40, 272, 378
Critical care
  Nursing practice   100
Diagnosis, radiologic   174
Digestion   40, 272
Diseases   415
Electrolyte disturbances
  74, 392
Endocrine system   40, 153,
  378, 405
  Gynecology   76
Fetus   318
Gastrointestinal system
  168, 169, 378
Genitourinary system   57
Genitourinary system, fe-
  male   191
Growth and development
  272
Gynecology   76, 106, 311
  Adolescence   186
  Nursing practice   258
Hematology   207
History and physical exam-
  ination   174
Human behavior   89
Initialisms   9
Kidneys   236
Liver   132
Metabolism   272, 378
Nervous system   92, 272,
  306, 378
  Nursing practice   63
Neural control systems   40
Newborns   318
  Nursing practice   258
Obstetrics   441
Ophthalmology   323
  Nursing practice   316

Orthopedics   327
Otolaryngology   328, 411
  Nursing practice   316
Pain
  Nervous system   306
Pathology
  Allergy   388
  Cardiorenal system   388
  Classification systems
    398
  Communicable diseases
    388
  Endocrine system   388
  Gastrointestinal system
    388
  Hematology   388
  Metabolism   388
  Respiratory system   388
  Rheumatology   388
  Toxicology   388
Pediatrics
  Gynecology   186
  Nursing practice   88
Pregnancy   441
  Complications   266
Renal failure   392
Respiratory system   40,
  272, 365, 378, 413
Rheumatology   31
Sensory systems   40
Sexual function, male   57
Sexuality   89
Symbols   378
Veterinary medicine
  Cats   416
  Dogs   416

PHYTIC ACID COMPOSITION

Foods   245

PIGS

  BT Animals
  Veterinary medicine
    Diseases
      Autopsies   432
      Control   432
      Diagnosis   432
      Etiology   432
      Pathogenesis   432
      Pathology   432
      Signs and symptoms
        432
      Treatment   432

UF-Used For, BT-Broader Term, NT-Narrower Term, RT-Related Term

PLACENTA

RT Pregnancy
Gynecology 310
Obstetrics 310

PLANT KINGDOM

RT Plants
Biology
Classification systems
209

PLANT SOURCES

Cosmetics
Natural ingredients
Encyclopedias 149
Drugs
Natural ingredients
Encyclopedias 149
Food products
Natural ingredients
Encyclopedias 149

PLANTS

NT Algae
NT Plants, medicinal
RT Botanicals
RT Plant kingdom
RT Strains, plant viruses
& antisera
Common names 48
Poisoning (of humans)
Classification systems
353
Common names 353
Diagnosis 193, 215,
351
Etiology 215
Geographic distribution
353
Illustrations 353
Lesions 353
Mechanisms of intoxica-
tion 353
Nursing practice 144
Pathophysiology 215
Physical descriptions
353
Prevention 193
Prognosis 193, 215
Scientific names 353
Signs and symptoms 193,
215, 351, 353

Toxicology 48, 353
Treatment 193, 215, 351
Scientific names 48

PLANTS, MEDICINAL

BT Plants
Atlases 247
Botanical names 247
Chemical constituents 247
Cultivation 247
Descriptions 247
Families 247
Former medicinal uses 247
Harvesting 247
Medicinal uses 247
Origin and distribution
247
Propagation 247
Synonyms 247
Toxicology 247

PLASTIC SURGERY

UF Reconstructive surgery
BT Treatment, surgical
Disability, physical 237
Otolaryngology
Techniques 328
Reconstruction
Anatomy 369
Classification systems
369
History 369
Preoperative examina-
tions 369
Techniques 369
Techniques 360
Head 411
Neck 411

PLEDGES (TEXTS)

American College of Physicians 45
American Psychiatry Asso-
ciation 44

PNEUMATIC COUNTER PRESSURE
DEVICE

RT Respiratory system
Techniques 115

POISON CONTROL CENTERS

RT   Health care services
RT   Poisoning
 Addresses   225, 246, 261,
  296, 348, 349
 Telephone numbers   5, 225,
  246, 261, 296, 348, 349

POISONING

NT   Food poisoning
RT   Bites and stings
RT   Emergency care
RT   Overdosage
RT   Poison control centers
RT   Toxicology
 Animals, marine
  Biology   352
  Chemistry   352
  Diagnosis   215
  Etiology   215
  Geographical distribu-
   tion   352
  Illustrations   352
  Intoxication mechanisms
   352
  Nomenclatures   352
  Pathology   352
  Pathophysiology   215
  Pharmacology   352
  Prevention   352
  Prognosis   215
  Signs and symptoms   215,
   352
  Treatment   215, 352
 Chemicals
  Diagnosis   193, 351
  Prevention   193
  Prognosis   193
  Signs and symptoms   193,
   351
  Treatment   193
 Commercial products, chem-
  icals
  Emergency treatment   85
  First aid   85
  Signs and symptoms   85
  Treatment   85
 Cosmetics
  Diagnosis   193, 351
  Prevention   193
  Prognosis   193
  Signs and symptoms   193,
   351
  Treatment   193, 351
 Critical care
  Nursing practice   100

 Diagnosis   360
  Adverse effects   105
 Drugs
  Diagnosis   193, 351
  Prevention   193
  Prognosis   193
  Signs and symptoms   193,
   351
  Treatment   138, 193, 351
 Drugs, new
  Treatment   138
 Emergency care
  Assessment, prehospital
   143
  Nursing practice   144
  Pathophysiology   143
  Signs and symptoms   143
  Stabilization, emergency
   room   143
 Family practice   281
 Household products
  Diagnosis   351
  Signs and symptoms   351
  Treatment   351
 Industrial hazards
  Diagnosis   351
  Signs and symptoms   351
  Treatment   351
 Insecticides
  Diagnosis   351
  Signs and symptoms   351
  Treatment   351
 Pediatrics
  Etiology   195
  Signs and symptoms   192,
   195, 304
  Treatment   108, 109,
   192, 195, 304
 Plants
  Classification systems
   353
  Common names   353
  Diagnosis   193, 215, 351
  Etiology   215
  Geographic distribution
   353
  Illustrations   353
  Lesions   353
  Mechanisms of intoxica-
   tion   353
  Nursing practice   144
  Pathophysiology   215
  Physical descriptions
   353
  Prevention   193
  Prognosis   193, 215

Scientific names 353
Signs and symptoms   193,
215, 351, 353
Toxicology 48, 353
Treatment   193, 215,
351
Prevention 351
Signs and symptoms 105,
111, 196, 286, 350, 351,
360
Snakebites
Diagnosis 215
Pathogenesis 215
Pathology 215
Prevention 215
Signs and symptoms 215
Treatment 215
Toxicology 351
Treatment 111, 196, 286,
350, 351, 356, 360
Adverse effects 105
Veterinary medicine
Small animals
Diagnosis 113
Prognosis 113
Signs and symptoms
113
Treatment 113

POLLUTION

See specific type

POLYGLOTS

RT Dictionaries
Medicine
English 141
French 141
German 141
Italian 141
Spanish 141

POLYPEPTIDES

RT Amino acids
RT Peptides
Biochemistry
Tabular data
Handbooks 94

POPLINE

BT Data bases
RT Data base access
Journals

Abbreviations 243
History 243
ISSN's 243
NLM call numbers 243

POPULATION

Statistical data 443

POSITIONS, ANATOMICAL

RT Anatomy
Orthopedics 254

POSTOPERATIVE CARE

See Treatment, surgical

POSTPARTUM PERIOD

RT Childbirth
RT Obstetrics
Nursing practice 258

PRACTICE MANAGEMENT

RT Family practice
Family medicine
Computers 406
Financial data 406
Medical records 406
Office design 406
Personnel 406

PREGNANCY

RT Abortion
RT Childbirth
RT Conception
RT Embryology
RT Gynecology
RT Obstetrics
RT Placenta
RT Reproduction
Adolescence 266
Anesthesia 28
Antepartal care
Nursing practice 258
Biophysical aspects
Nursing practice 258
Complications 191, 266,
318, 441
Biochemistry 266
Drug abuse 266
Nursing practice 258
Pathology 310

Physiology 266
Signs and symptoms 266
Treatment 266
Diagnosis 191
Animals 146
Drugs 20, 188, 296, 427, 428
Nursing practice 137, 312
Embryo development
Nursing practice 258
Embryo physiology
Nursing practice 258
Emotional aspects 191
Endocrine system 405
Gynecology 76
Fetus development
Nursing practice 258
Fetus physiology
Nursing practice 258
High risk patients 266
Home delivery 191
Hypertension 78, 266, 372
Nutrition 293
Nursing practice 258
Parent education
Nursing practice 258
Patient education
Guides 21
Physiology 441
Postpartum period
Nursing practice 258
Prenatal care 191
Psychosocial aspects
Nursing practice 258
Puerperium 318
Renal function 372
Risk factors
Nursing practice 258
Sexuality
Nursing practice 214

PREMEDICAL PROGRAMS

RT Medical schools
Ratings
Undergraduate schools
177

PRENATAL CARE

See Fetus

PREOPERATIVE CARE

See Treatment, surgical

PREVENTION

RT Chemoprophylaxis
RT Immunizations
RT Preventive medicine
Accidents 259
Adverse effects
Anesthesia, regional 238
Athletic injuries 419
Diseases
Cancer 61, 259
Communicable diseases 91, 223, 259, 355
Tropical medicine 215
Dentistry 5, 259
Dermatology 116
Environmental diseases 259
Family practice 281
Heart 259
Immunology 37
Kidneys 259
Mental illness 259
Mental retardation 259
Nosocomial infections 259, 355
Nutrition 293
Nutritional deficiencies
Tropical medicine 215
Occupational diseases 319
Ophthalmology 171
Parasitology
Arthropods 83
Helminths 83
Protozoa 83
Pediatrics 304, 339
Poisoning 351
Animals, marine 352
Bites and stings 193
Cosmetics 193
Drugs 193
Foods 193, 259
Plants 193
Snakebites 215
Sexually transmitted diseases 259
Tropical medicine 215

PREVENTIVE MEDICINE

RT Prevention
Encyclopedias, loose-leaf 81
Nursing practice

Information sources   303

PRICES

UF   Cost
RT   Charges
RT   Fees
Books, in print   53
Drug store merchandise
Biologicals   136
Botanicals   136
Cosmetics   136
Drugs   19, 136
Fountain products   136
Perfumes   136
Pharmaceuticals   136
Stationery   136
Medical devices   267

PROBABILITY

RT   Statistical data
CRC handbooks
Indexes   93
Tabular data   170

PROBLEM-ORIENTED MEDICAL RE-
CORDS

BT   Medical records
History and physical examination   181

PROCEDURES

See also specific subjects
UF   Techniques
Classification systems
Anesthesiology   347
Diagnosis, radiologic
347
Laboratory medicine   347
Medicine   347
Pathology   347
Treatment, surgical   347

PROCEEDINGS, PUBLISHED

RT   Meetings, past
Bibliographies   127, 221,
361
Journal sources   444
Ordering information   127,
221

PRODUCTS, MEDICAL, MANUFAC-

TURERS

See Manufacturers, medical
products

PROGNOSIS

Diseases
Ambulatory medicine   358
Birth defects   49
Cancer   7, 60
Communicable diseases
223, 355
Pediatrics   224
Treatment, surgical
395
Tropical medicine   215
Dermatology   116
Genetics   270
Genitourinary system
172
Gynecology   191
Handbooks   105, 286, 356
Hematology   207
Immunology   37
Liver   133
Mouth   410
Nervous system   306
Nursing practice   63
Newborns   382
Nutritional deficiencies
215
Ophthalmology   171
Orthopedics   327
Parasitology
Arthropods   83
Helminths   83
Protozoa   83
Patient education   21
Pediatrics   108, 192,
304, 339
Hematology   208
Poisoning
Bites and stings   193
Chemicals   193
Cosmetics   193
Drugs   193
Fish
Tropical medicine
215
Foods   193
Plants   193
Tropical medicine
215
Veterinary medicine
Small animals   113

Respiratory system   365
Syndromes   121
Treatment, surgical   110

PRONUNCIATION

Drugs   280, 429
Nursing practice   137
Patient education   427

PROOFREADING MARKS

RT   Authors' guides
RT   Writing, medical
Manuals   249

PROPRIETARY NAMES

See Brand names

PROTEINS

NT   Enzymes
RT   Amino acids
RT   Peptides
Biochemistry   43
Tabular data   94
Microbial composition
Tabular data   98

PROTOCOLS, CANCER

See Cancer protocols, ex-
perimental

PROTOZOA

RT   Parasitology
RT   Strains, protozoa
Biology   83
Classification systems
83
Diagnosis, immunologic
83
Diseases
Diagnosis   83
Epidemiology   83
Pathogenesis   83
Pathology   83
Prevention   83
Prognosis   83
Signs and symptoms   83
Treatment   83
Etomologic methods   83
History   83
Illustrations   83

Life cycles   83
Morphology   83
Specimen examination
techniques   83
Tabular data   98

PRURITUS

Differential diagnosis
244

PSYCHIATRIC MANIFESTATIONS

Diseases   291

PSYCHIATRIC SERVICES

Hospitals
Statistical data   212

PSYCHIATRISTS

See American Psychiatry
Association

PSYCHIATRY

BT   Behavioral sciences
NT   Child psychiatry
NT   Forensic psychiatry
RT   Mental illness
Dictionaries   364
Diseases
Case studies   291
Classification systems
89
Diagnosis   89, 291
Drugs (treatment modali-
ty)   89, 189, 291
Epidemiology   89
Etiology   89
Residential care   89
Signs and symptoms   89,
291
Treatment   89, 291
Drug abuse   291
Diagnosis   89
Signs and symptoms   89
Treatment   89
Emergencies
Diagnosis   89
Treatment   89
Encyclopedias, loose-leaf
81, 384
Glossaries   89
History   89, 291

Human behavior 89
Legal aspects 291
Mental retardation 291
Patient examination 291
Personality development
  291
Psychotherapy 89, 291
Shock treatment 291
Tests
  Nervous system 82
  Pediatrics 195

PUBLIC HEALTH

RT   Communicable diseases
RT   Public health schools
RT   Public health scien-
       tists
Accidents
  Epidemiology 259
  Prevention 259
Behavioral factors
  Alcohol use 259
  Drug use 259
  Lifestyles 259
  Smoking tobacco 259
Cancer
  Epidemiology 259
  Prevention 259
Cardiovascular system
  Diseases
    Epidemiology 259
    Prevention 259
Communicable diseases
  Complications 259
  Control 259
  Diagnosis 259
  Epidemiology 259
  Etiology 259
  History 259
  Immunology 259
  Occurrence 259
  Pathology 259
  Prevention 259
  Signs and symptoms 259
  Transmission 259
  Treatment 259
Dentistry
  Diseases
    Epidemiology 259
    Prevention 259
Environmental diseases
  Prevention 259
  Signs and symptoms 259
Food poisoning
  Complications 259

Control 259
Diagnosis 259
Epidemiology 259
Etiology 259
History 259
Immunology 259
Occurrence 259
Pathology 259
Prevention 259
Signs and symptoms 259
Transmission 259
Treatment 259
Kidneys
  Diseases
    Epidemiology 259
    Prevention 259
Mental illness
  Epidemiology 259
  Prevention 259
Mental retardation
  Epidemiology 259
  Prevention 259
Nosocomial infections
  Complications 259
  Control 259
  Diagnosis 259
  Epidemiology 259
  Etiology 259
  History 259
  Immunology 259
  Occurrence 259
  Pathology 259
  Prevention 259
  Signs and symptoms 259
  Transmission 259
  Treatment 259
Nutrition 259
Occupational health
  Regulations 259
Sexually transmitted dis-
  eases
  Complications 259
  Control 259
  Diagnosis 259
  Epidemiology 259
  Etiology 259
  History 259
  Immunology 259
  Occurrence 259
  Pathology 259
  Prevention 259
  Signs and symptoms 259
  Transmission 259
  Treatment 259
Solid waste disposal 259
Water quality management

259

PUBLIC HEALTH SCHOOLS

UF   Education, public
       health schools
BT   University programs
RT   Public health
 Directories
    Addresses   46, 341
    Chairpersons   341
    Deans   46
    Expenses   341
    Faculty, number of   341
    Programs offered   341
    Students, number of   341
    Telephone numbers   341
    University community
    341
 Ratings
    Graduate schools   176

PUBLIC HEALTH SCIENTISTS

BT   Scientists
RT   Public health
 Directories
    Addresses   23
    Birth dates   23
    Educational backgrounds
    23
    Marriage dates   23
    Memberships   23
    Professional experience
    23
    Specialties   23

PUBLIC RELATIONS

 Health care
    Directories   381

PUBLICATIONS

NT   Books
NT   Journals
 Archives   129
 Information centers   129
 Information services   150
 Information systems   150
 Libraries, research   129
 Libraries, special   129
 Organizations   147, 198,
    261, 385, 446
 Research centers   375
 Research institutes, for-

eign   445

PUBLISHERS

 Books   381
    Addresses   53, 265
    Telephone numbers   53,
    265
 Journals
    Addresses   102, 103,
    265, 420
    Telephone numbers   420
 Proceedings   127

PUBLISHING, MEDICAL

RT   Authors' guides
 Style manuals   213, 249
 Writing techniques   213

PUERPERIUM

RT   Childbirth
RT   Obstetrics
 Pregnancy   318

PULMONARY FUNCTION TESTING

RT   Respiratory system
 Anesthesia practice, con-
    sultant
    Techniques   27

PULMONARY MANIFESTATIONS

 Systemic diseases   413

PULMONARY MEDICINE

 See Respiratory system

PULP PROTECTION

RT   Dentistry
 Dentistry, operative   320

PURINES

RT   Nutrition
 Biochemistry
    Tabular data   94

PYRIMIDINES

 Biochemistry
    Tabular data   94

UF–Used For, BT–Broader Term, NT–Narrower Term, RT–Related Term

QUALITY ASSURANCE STANDARDS

UF   Standards
RT   Joint Commission on Ac-
     creditation of Hospi-
     tals
  Hospitals
    Diseases
      Charges 332
      Indications for admis-
      sion 332
      Indications for diag-
      nostic tests 332
      Indications for dis-
      charge 332
      Indications for treat-
      ment 332
      Length of stay 332

QUOTATIONS

  Dictionaries
    Medicine 161

RADIATION POLLUTION

  RT   Air pollution
  RT   Ecology
  RT   Environmental health
    Chemical materials, indus-
    trial
      Control 114
      Hazards 114

RADIATION THERAPY

  See Treatment, radiation

RADIOACTIVE NUCLIDES

  RT   Diagnosis, radiologic
    CRC handbooks
      Indexes 93

RADIOGRAPHIC ANATOMY

  RT   Diagnosis, radiologic
    Head
      Atlases 32
    Neck
      Atlases 32

RADIOISOTOPES

  RT   Diagnosis, radiologic
    Pharmaceutical practice

     371
    Tabular data 285

RADIOLOGIC DIAGNOSIS

  See Diagnosis, radiologic

RADIOLOGIC TECHNOLOGY

  RT   Diagnosis, radiologic
    Indexes, literature 315

RAPE

  BT   Sexual assault
    Medicolegal investigations
    292

RATINGS

    Graduate schools 176
    Undergraduate schools 177

REAGENTS

  UF   Test reagents
  RT   Chemistry
  RT   Laboratory science,
       clinical
    Catalogs
      Ordering information
        Characteristics 307
        Classification systems
        307
        Cultures 307
        Potencies 307
        Producers 307
        Purity 307
        Strains 307
    Chemicals, European 155
    Diagnosis, laboratory
      Bacteriology 179
      Hematology 207, 240
    Microbiology
      Formulas 35
      Procedures 35

RECOMMENDED DIETARY ALLOW-
ANCES

  RT   Foods
  RT   Nutrition
    Tabular data 54, 145, 400

RECONSTRUCTIVE SURGERY

See Plastic surgery

RECTAL SUPPOSITORIES

BT Drugs
Patient education   280

RECTUM

BT Alimentary tract
BT Gastrointestinal system
Diseases
  Signs and symptoms   394
  Treatment, surgical
    Techniques   393, 394

REFERENCE BOOKS

BT Books
Bibliographies, annotated
182
Allied health sciences
201
Medicine   201, 273
Veterinary medicine   201
Core collection
Indexes, thesauri   162
Toxicology
Information sources   225

REFERENCE STANDARDS

Drugs   426

REGISTRY NUMBERS, CAS

See CAS registry numbers

REHABILITATION

RT Occupational therapy
RT Physical therapy
Athletic injuries   419
Disability, physical   237
Diseases
  Cancer   61
  Nervous system
    Encyclopedias, loose-
      leaf   82
  Rheumatology   414
Indexes, literature   315

RENAL

See Kidneys

RENAL MANIFESTATIONS

Systemic diseases   392

REPRODUCTION

RT Conception
RT Gynecology
RT Obstetrics
RT Pregnancy
Biology
  Tabular data   48
Endocrine system   153
Laboratory animal sciences
Handbooks   97

RESEARCH AWARDS, HEALTH

See Health research awards

RESEARCH CENTERS

NT Cancer research insti-
    tutes
RT Libraries, research
    centers
Directories   381
Addresses   375
Dates founded   375
Directors   375
Facilities   375
Financial data   375
Library facilities   375
Parent institutions   375
Publications   375
Research activities   375
Staff, number of   375
Support sources   375
Telephone numbers   375

RESEARCH INSTITUTES, FOREIGN

RT Cancer research insti-
    tutes
Directories
Addresses   445
Officials   445
Publications   445
Telephone numbers   445

RESEARCH LIBRARIES

See Libraries, research

RESEARCH PROGRAMS

UF-Used For, BT-Broader Term, NT-Narrower Term, RT-Related Term

RT   Cancer research insti-
       tutes
RT   Health research awards
Directories
   Allied health sciences
      Addresses   376
      Cable addresses   376
      Officials   376
      Research activities
         376
      Staff, number of   376
      Telephone numbers   376
      Telex numbers   376
      TWX numbers   376
   Biomedical sciences
      Addresses   376
      Cable addresses   376
      Officials   376
      Research activities
         376
      Staff, number of   376
      Telephone numbers   376
      Telex numbers   376
      TWX numbers   376
   Dentistry
      Addresses   376
      Cable addresses   376
      Officials   376
      Research activities
         376
      Staff, number of   376
      Telephone numbers   376
      Telex numbers   376
      TWX numbers   376
   Medical sciences
      Addresses   376
      Cable addresses   376
      Officials   376
      Research activities
         376
      Staff, number of   376
      Telephone numbers   376
      Telex numbers   376
      TWX numbers   376
   Pharmacology
      Addresses   376
      Cable addresses   376
      Officials   376
      Research activities
         376
      Staff, number of   376
      Telephone numbers   376
      Telex numbers   376
      TWX numbers   376
   Veterinary medicine
      Addresses   376

      Cable addresses   376
      Officials   376
      Research activities
         376
      Staff, number of   376
      Telephone numbers   376
      Telex numbers   376
      TWX numbers   376

RESIDENCY PROGRAMS, ACCREDI-
TED

   RT   Medical schools
   Directories
      Addresses   128
      Admissions, annual   128
      Advertisements   178
      Affiliations, medical
         schools   128
      Autopsies, percentage of
         128
      Beds, number of   128
      Census, average daily
         128
      Housing   178
      Medical education direc-
         tors   128
      Medical staff, number in
         128
      Photographs   178
      Program directors   128
      Salaries   178
   Specialty requirements
      128
   Statistical data   128, 178

RESPIRATION

   RT   Respiratory system
   Biology
      Tabular data   48
   Pathophysiology   331
   Physiology   40, 272, 378

RESPIRATORY CARE

   RT   Respiratory system
   Anesthesia practice, con-
      sultant
      Techniques   27
   Pediatrics
      Treatment, surgical   397

RESPIRATORY SYSTEM

   UF   Lungs

UF   Pulmonary medicine
RT   Pneumatic counter pres-
     sure device
RT   Pulmonary function
     testing
RT   Respiration
RT   Respiratory care
RT   Respiratory therapy
RT   Thorax
 Acid-base balance   117
 Anatomy   117, 365
 Biochemistry   413
 Blood gases   117
 Chest roentgen screening
 117
 Diagnosis
   Techniques   117, 413
 Differential diagnosis
   Decision trees   117
 Diseases
   Diagnosis   173, 365,
     366, 413
   Diagnosis, radiologic
   117
   Etiology   117, 365, 413
   Pathogenesis   117, 413
   Pathology   117, 365
   Physiology   413
   Prognosis   365
   Signs and symptoms   117,
     365, 366
   Treatment   173, 365,
     366, 413
   Treatment, surgical   173
 Encyclopedias, loose-leaf
 81, 384
 History and physical exam-
   ination   117
 Immunology   413
 Lung biopsies   117
 Morphology   413
 Pathology
   Physiology   388
 Physiology   117, 365, 413
 Pulmonary circulation
   Diseases
     Diagnosis   365
     Pathology   365
     Physiology   365
     Prognosis   365
     Signs and symptoms
     365
     Treatment   365
 Pulmonary manifestations
   Systemic diseases   413
 Ultrasonography   117

RESPIRATORY THERAPY

   RT   Respiratory system
   Indexes, literature   315

RESTORATIONS

   Dentistry, operative   320

RESUMES

   RT   Job hunting
   Examples   362
   Guidelines   362
   Manuals   362

RESUSCITATION

   See Cardiopulmonary resuscitation

REVIEW ARTICLES

   RT   Indexes, literature
   Behavioral sciences   222
   Biomedicine   218
   Medicine   218, 222

RH ISOIMMUNIZATION

   Immunizations   37

RHEUMATOLOGY

   UF   Arthritis
   Anatomy   31
   Diagnosis
     Techniques   414
   Diseases
     Diagnosis   31, 84, 414
     Diagnosis, radiologic
     31
     Differential diagnosis
     31, 84, 414
     Drugs (treatment modali-
     ty)   84
       Adverse effects   31,
       414
       Dosage and administra-
       tion   31, 414
       Indications   31, 414
       Pharmacokinetics   31,
       414
       Toxicology   31, 414
     Epidemiology   31
     Etiology   31, 414

Examination 84
Immunopathology 31
Occupational therapy 84
Pathogenesis 31
Pathology 31, 414
Pathophysiology 31
Physical therapy 84
Rehabilitation 414
Signs and symptoms 31,
  84, 414
Treatment 31, 84, 414
Encyclopedias, loose-leaf
  81, 384
History and physical exam-
  ination 414
Immunology 414
Inflammatory process 414
Metabolism 414
Pathology
  Physiology 388
Physiology 31

RICKETTSIAE

RT   Bacteriology
RT   Communicable diseases
RT   Spirochetes
RT   Strains, rickettsiae
  Microbiology
    Assays 251
    Characterization 251
    Culture and isolation
      251
    Examination 251
    Identifications 251
    Interpretations 251
    Serodiagnosis 251
    Tests 251

RICKETTSIOLOGY

  Laboratory science, clinical
    Tabular data 99

RIGHTS OF PATIENTS

  See Patient rights

RISK FACTORS

  Cancer (in U.S.)
    Statisical data 59
  Pregnancy
    Nursing practice 258

ROUTES OF ADMINISTRATION
(DRUGS)

  See Dosage and administration

RUNAWAY YOUTH CENTERS

  RT   Health care services
  RT   Pediatrics
    Directories 203
      Addresses 297
      Contact persons 297
      Telephone numbers 297

SALARIES

  RT   Incomes, net
    Hospitals
      Nursing practice 317
      Residency training pro-
      grams 178

SCHOLARSHIPS

  RT   Financial aid
    Nursing
      Information sources 303

SCHOOLS

  See Education for specific
  types

SCIENCES

  See also specific science
    Abbreviations 9
    Acronyms 9
    Directories
      Bibliographies 124
    Indexes, citations 383
    Indexes, literature
      Review articles 222
    Initialisms 9
    Journals
      Abbreviations 340
    Meetings
      Proceedings, published
      127, 221, 361, 444

SCIENTIFIC NAMES

  UF   Names, scientific
    Animals 48
    Plants 48

Poisoning   353

SCIENTIFIC ORGANIZATIONS

See Organizations,
scientific

SCIENTIFIC TABLES

CRC handbooks
Indexes   93

SCIENTISTS

NT   Biological scientists
NT   Public health scien-
tists
Directories
Addresses   23
Birth dates   23
Educational backgrounds
23
Marriage dates   23
Memberships   23
Professional experience
23
Specialties   23

SCREENING

Birth defects
Pediatrics   339

SEASONAL DISTRIBUTIONS

Morbidity
Communicable diseases
Statistical data   443

SECRETARY OF HEALTH & HUMAN
SERVICES

Annual reports
Health status   204
Health trends   204

SELECTION FACTORS

Dental schools   10
Medical schools   275

SELF-MEDICATION GUIDELINES

Drugs, nonprescription
190

SELF-TREATMENT

Patient education   349

SENATORS AND REPRESENTATIVES

RT   Congressional subcom-
mittees
Directories
Addresses   299
Aides, health issues
299
Appointment secretaries
299
District offices
Addresses   299
Contact persons   299
Telephone numbers   299
Health committee member-
ship   299
Health subcommittee mem-
bership   299
Telephone numbers   299

SENSORY SYSTEMS

Physiology   40

SERIALS

See Journals

SERODIAGNOSIS

BT   Diagnosis
RT   Blood
RT   Hematology
Communicable diseases
Interpretations of
tests   179
Laboratory techniques
179
Microbiology
Bacteriology   251
Fungi   251
Parasitology   251
Rickettsiae   251
Spirochetes   251
Techniques   35
Viruses   251

SERVICES

NT   Health care services
Classification systems
Anesthesiology   347

UF-Used For, BT-Broader Term, NT-Narrower Term, RT-Related Term

Diagnosis, radiologic
  347
Laboratory medicine   347
Medicine   347
Pathology   347
Treatment, surgical   347

SEX COUNSELING

  BT   Counseling services
  Directories   381
  Nursing practice   258

SEX DIFFERENTIATION

  Endocrine system   153, 405

SEX EDUCATION

  Directories   381
  Gynecology   311

SEX RATIO

  Mental disorders   118

SEXES

  Deaths
    Statistical data   443
  Morbidity
    Communicable diseases
      Statistical data   443

SEXUAL ASSAULT

  NT   Rape
  Nursing practice   214

SEXUAL FUNCTION, MALE

  RT   Sexuality
  Infertility
    Etiology   57
    Treatment   57
  Physiology   57

SEXUALITY

  RT   Gynecology
  RT   Sexual function, male
  Abortion
    Psychological aspects
    89
    Techniques   89
  Adolescence   109

Gynecology   186
Aged   72
Anatomy   89
Coitus techniques   89
Contraception
  Psychological aspects
  89
  Techniques   89
Diseases   89
Endocrine system   89
  Gynecology   76
Family practice
  Handbooks   281
Gynecology   106
Nursing practice
  Abortion   214
  Assessment   214
  Contraception   214
  Disease states   214
  Drug effects   214
  Dysfunction
    Etiology   214
    Treatment   214
  Infertility   214
  Life cycle   214
  Pregnancy   214
  Sexual assault   214
  Sexual response   258
  Sexually transmitted
    diseases   214
Patient education   21
Pediatrics
  Gynecology   186
Physiology   89
Psychosomatic disorders
  Signs and symptoms   89
  Treatment   89

SEXUALLY TRANSMITTED DISEASES

  BT   Communicable diseases
  Public health
    Complications   259
    Control   259
    Diagnosis   259
    Public health   259
    Epidemiology   259
    Etiology   259
    History   259
    Immunology   259
    Occurrence   259
    Pathology   259
    Prevention   259
    Sexuality   214
    Signs and symptoms   259
    Transmission   259

Treatment   259

SHEEP

BT Animals
Veterinary medicine
Diseases
Autopsies   432
Control   432
Diagnosis   432
Etiology   432
Pathogenesis   432
Pathology   432
Signs and symptoms   432
Treatment   432

SHOCK

Emergency care   136
Nursing practice
Assessment   144
Complications   144
Etiology   144
Pathology   144
Pathophysiology   144
Signs and symptoms
144
Treatment   144
Psychiatry   291
Treatment, surgical   4,
110, 360

SIGN LANGUAGE

RT Deaf services
RT Handicapped services
Dentistry   276
Emergency care   276
First aid   276
Medicine   276

SIGNS AND SYMPTOMS

UF Symptoms
RT Differential diagnosis
RT Systemic diseases
Accidents   286
Air pollution
Toxicology   175
Birth defects   49
Bites and stings   193, 196,
351
Emergency care
Nursing practice   144
Handbooks   111
Pediatrics   304

Poisoning   351
Tabular data   286
Burns
Handbooks   111
Chemicals
Poisoning   193, 351
Commercial products, chem-
icals
Poisoning   85
Toxicology   85
Cosmetics
Poisoning   193, 351
Diseases   38, 67, 73, 145,
181, 288, 329, 356, 360,
415
Abdomen   4
Acid-base disturbances
236
Nursing practice   314
Adolescence
Gynecology   186
Adrenals   57
Allergy   12
Ambulatory medicine   358
Anus   394
Bile ducts   132, 133
Blood vessels   205
Body fluid disturbances
236
Nursing practice   314
Cancer   7, 60
Child psychiatry   89
Colon   394
Communicable diseases
223, 296, 355
Pediatrics   224, 296
Public health   259
Treatment, surgical
395
Tropical medicine   215
Dermatology   26, 116
Dictionaries   50, 217
Differential diagnosis
166
Anemia   244
Bleeding   244
Coma   244
Constipation   244
Convulsions   244
Cough   244
Cyanosis   244
Dehydration   244
Diarrhea   244
Dizziness   244
Dyspnea   244
Edema   244

UF-Used For, BT-Broader Term, NT-Narrower Term, RT-Related Term

Fatigue 244
Fever 244
Headache 244
Hypertension 244
Jaundice 244
Nausea 244
Nervousness 244
Obesity 244
Pain 244
Pallor 244
Pruritus 244
Skin color 244
Syncope 244
Undernutrition 244
Vertigo 244
Electrolyte disturbances
236, 372, 392
  Nursing practice 314
Emergency care 143, 253
  Pediatrics 143, 192,
  252, 412
Encyclopedias 196
Encyclopedias, loose-
  leaf 81
Endocrine system 153,
405
Environmental diseases
259
Family medicine 281,
406
Gallbladder 132, 133
Gastrointestinal system
75, 168, 169
Genetics 270, 284, 287
Genitourinary system
172
Genitourinary system,
  female 185
Gynecology 106, 191,
310, 311, 318
Handbooks 104, 105,
111, 190, 253, 286
  Pediatrics 192, 439
Heart 205, 206
Hematology 77, 207, 240
  Pediatrics 208
Hypertension 78
Immunology 37
Kidneys 236, 372, 392
Liver 132, 133
Malnutrition 293
Mendelian inheritance
  Genetics 284
Mental illness 89, 118,
291
Metabolism 368

Mouth 324, 410
Nervous system 359, 408
  Encyclopedias, loose-
  leaf 82
  Handbooks 92
Neuro-ophthalmology 171
Newborns 382
Nosocomial infections
  Public health 259
Nursing practice 242,
277, 333
Nutritional deficiencies
293
  Tropical medicine 215
  Vitamins 175
Obstetrics 310
Occupational diseases
  Indexes 220
Ophthalmology 171, 323
  Nursing practice 316
Orthopedics 326
Otolaryngology 328
  Nursing practice 316
Parasitology
  Arthropods 83
  Helminths 83
  Protozoa 83
Patient education
  Guides 21
Pediatrics 108, 304,
339
  Communicable diseases
  224, 296
  Emergency care 252
  Gastrointestinal sys-
  tem 335
  Gynecology 186
  Handbooks 192, 439
  Hematology 208
  Nursing practice 88
  Ophthalmology 336
  Orthopedics 337
Pregnancy 266
  Nursing practice
  Maternity care 258
Psychiatry 89, 118, 291
Rectum 394
Respiratory system 117,
365, 366
Rheumatology 31, 84,
414
Sexually transmitted
diseases
  Public health 259
Treatment, surgical
  Handbooks 110

Nursing practice
  Patient care   277
Urology   57
  Handbooks   112
Veterinary medicine   51
  Cats   416
  Cattle   432
  Dogs   416
  Horses   432
  Pigs   432
  Sheep   432
  Small animals
Drug abuse
  Nervous system
    Encyclopedias, loose-
      leaf   82
  Psychiatry   89
Drugs
  Poisoning   193, 351
Fish
  Poisoning
    Tropical medicine   215
Industrial hazards
  Poisoning   351
Injuries   286
Insecticides
  Poisoning   351
Overdose
  Drugs, nonprescription
    349
Pesticides
  Toxicology   175
Poisoning   351, 360
  Adverse effects   105
  Animals   351
  Animals, marine   352
  Chemicals   193, 351
    Commercial products
    85
  Cosmetics   193, 351
  Diagnosis   360
  Drugs   193, 351
  Emergency care   143
  Encyclopedias   196
  Fish   215
  Food poisoning   168, 193
    Nursing practice   144
    Public health   259
  Handbooks   111, 350
  Household products   351
  Industrial hazards   351
  Insecticides   351
  Pediatrics   304
    Handbooks   192, 195
  Pesticides   175
  Plants   193, 351, 353

Nursing practice   144
  Tropical medicine   215
Small animals
  Veterinary medicine
  113
Snakebites
  Tropical medicine   215
Solvents   175
Tabular data   286
Treatment   360
Psychosomatic disorders
  Sexuality   89
Snakebites
  Poisoning
    Tropical medicine   215
Solvents
  Toxicology   175
Syndromes   121, 368
  Chromosomal anomalies
    69
  Dictionaries   217
Toxicology   67
Trauma
  Emergency care   143
    Nursing practice   144
  Nervous system   306

SINGLE ADULTS

  Family medicine   406

SKIN

  See Dermatology

SKIN DISEASES

  See Dermatology

SKIN GRAFTING

  RT Dermatology
    Orthopedics   326

SKIN MANIFESTATIONS

  RT Dermatology
    Differential diagnosis
    244
    Systemic diseases   116

SLIDES

  See Audiovisual materials

SMALL ANIMALS

UF-Used For, BT-Broader Term, NT-Narrower Term, RT-Related Term

NT Cats
NT Dogs
  Veterinary medicine
    Cats
      Normal laboratory
        values 113
      Diseases
        Diagnosis 113
        Etiology 113
        Pathophysiology 113
        Prognosis 113
        Signs and symptoms
          113
        Treatment 113
    Dogs
      Normal laboratory
        values 113
      Poisoning
        Diagnosis 113
        Prognosis 113
        Signs and symptoms
          113
        Treatment 113

SMOKING CESSATION PROGRAMS

  Health care services
    Directories 203

SMOKING (TOBACCO)

  UF Cigarette smoking
  Behavioral factors
    Public health 259

SNAKEBITES

  BT Bites and stings
  Poisoning
    Tropical medicine
      Diagnosis 215
      Pathogenesis 215
      Pathology 215
      Prevention 215
      Signs and symptoms
        215
      Treatment 215

SOLID WASTE DISPOSAL

  Public health 259

SOLID WASTES

  Chemical materials, indus-
    trial

Control 114
Hazards 114

SOLUBILITY

  Drugs 371, 426
  Drugs, British 55

SOLVENTS

  BT Chemicals
  Toxicology
    Pharmacology 175
    Signs and symptoms 175
    Treatment 175

SPANISH

  Medicine
    Polyglots 141

SPECIAL COLLECTIONS

  Archives 129
  Information centers 129
  Libraries, research 129
  Libraries, special 129

SPECIAL LIBRARIES

  See Libraries, special

SPECIALISTS

  RT American specialty
        boards
  RT Physicians
  Biological scientists 23
  Members
    American College of Phy-
      sicians 45
    American College of Sur-
      geons 16
  Physical scientists 23
  Physicians 22, 126, 424
    Statistical data 346
  Physicians, women 130
  Public health scientists
    23
  Specialty requirements
    Residency programs, ac-
      credited 128

SPEECH DISORDERS

  RT Handicapped services

Pediatrics
Diagnosis   411

SPEECH PATHOLOGY

Ratings
Undergraduate schools
177

SPIDERS

See Arthropods

SPIROCHETES

RT   Bacteriology
RT   Rickettsiae
Microbiology
Assays   251
Characterization   251
Culture and isolation
251
Examination   251
Identifications   251
Interpretations   251
Serodiagnosis   251
Tests   251

SPLEEN

RT   Blood
RT   Hematology
Diseases
Treatment, surgical   393

SPORTS INJURIES

See Athletic injuries

STABILITY

Drugs   20
Drugs, injectable   194

STAGING

Cancer   61

STAINING TECHNIQUES

Bacteriology
Diagnosis, laboratory
179

STAINS

RT   Microbiology
Formulas
Diagnosis, laboratory
Bacteriology   179
Microbiology
Formulas   35
Procedures   35

STANDARDS

See Quality assurance
standards

STATE HEALTH OFFICES

Nursing
Directories   303

STATIONERY

Prices (retail & whole-
sale)
Catalogs
Drug store merchandise
136

STATISTICAL DATA

NT   Vital statistics
RT   Almanacs
RT   Handbooks
RT   Probability
RT   Tabular data
Allied health education
programs   13
Burn beds, number of
Burn centers   296
Cancer   296
Etiology   59
Incidence   59
Mortality   59
Research   59
Risk factors   59
Survival   59
Trends   59
Communicable diseases
Morbidity
Ages   443
Seasonal variations
443
Sexes   443
Death and dying   389
Diseases
Information sources   159
Divorce   436, 437
Fertility   204

UF-Used For, BT-Broader Term, NT-Narrower Term, RT-Related Term

Health care   58, 199, 436
  Health care expenditures
    157, 204
  Health care resources
    Utilization   157, 204
  Health status determi-
    nants   204
  Information sources   159
  Mortality   204
  Personnel
    Midwives, number of
      443
    Nurses, number of   443
    Physicians, number of
      443
Holdings
  Archives   129
  Information centers   129
  Libraries, medical   125
  Libraries, research   129
  Libraries, special   129
Hospitals
  Admission statistics
    184, 212
  Bassinets, number of
    184
  Beds, number of   128,
    184, 212, 317, 424
  Births, number of   184
  Census, average daily
    128, 184, 212
  Financial data   184, 212
  Occupancy, percentage
    184, 212
  Outpatient visits   212
  Payroll   212
  Personnel, number of
    184, 212
  Psychiatric services
    212
  Services   212, 424
  Utilization   212
Hospitals, Canada
  Admission statistics   58
  Beds, number of   58
  Births, number of   58
  Financial data   58
Hospitals, United Kingdom
  Beds, number of   268
Hospitals, world
  Admission statistics
    443
  Beds, number of   443
  Discharges, number of
    443
  Inpatient days, number

  of   443
Information sources   390
Licensure   425
  Dentistry   17
Manpower   199
Marriage   436, 437
Medical schools   275
Mortality   204, 389, 436
  Ages   443
  Causes of death   437,
    443
  Characteristics   437
  Rates   437
  Sexes   443
Mortality, accidents
  Causes of death   437
  Characteristics   437
  Rates   437
Mortality, fetal
  Causes of death   437
  Characteristics   437
  Rates   437
Mortality, infants
  Causes of death   437,
    443
  Characteristics   437
  Rates   437
Natality   436
  Characteristics   437
  Rates   437
Nurses
  Distribution   157
  Economic status   157
  Education   157
  Number of   443
Nursing education
  Accreditation   308
  Admissions   308
  Employment information
    308
  Enrollments   308
  Graduation   308
  Minority students   308
  Personal information
    308
  Programs   308
  Tuitions   308
Patients
  Health facilities   199
  Visits   363
Physicians
  Fees   363
  Geographic distribution
    346
  Incomes, net   363
  Number of   443

Personal characteristics
346
Professional activities
346
Professional expenses
363
Specialties 346
Work patterns 363
Residency programs, ac-
credited 128, 178
Vital statistics 436
Information sources 390
Population 443

STERILIZATION

RT Contraception
Obstetrics
Indications 191
Techniques 191
Pharmaceutical practice
371

STEROIDS

RT Endocrine system
RT Hormones
Biochemistry
Tabular data 94

STOMACH

BT Alimentary tract
BT Gastrointestinal system
Diseases
Treatment, surgical 393

STRAINS

RT Bacteriology
Medical firsts
Bibliographies 152
Ordering information
Reagents
Catalog 307
Original articles
Bibliographies 152

STRAINS, ALGAE

RT Algae
Descriptions
Catalogs
Cultures 65

STRAINS, ANIMAL VIRUSES

Descriptions
Catalogs
Cultures 66

STRAINS, BACTERIA

RT Bacteriology
Descriptions
Catalogs 39
Cultures 65

STRAINS, BACTERIOPHAGES

Descriptions
Catalogs
Cultures 65

STRAINS, CHLAMYDIAE

UF Chlamydiae
Descriptions
Catalogs
Cultures 66

STRAINS, FUNGI

RT Fungi
RT Mycology
Descriptions
Catalogs
Cultures 65

STRAINS, MYCOVIRUSES

UF Mycoviruses
Descriptions
Catalogs
Cultures 65

STRAINS, PLANT VIRUSES &
ANTISERA

RT Plants
Descriptions
Catalogs
Cultures 65

STRAINS, PROTOZOA

RT Protozoa
Descriptions
Catalogs
Cultures 65

STRAINS, RECOMBINANT DNA VEC-
TORS

UF—Used For, BT—Broader Term, NT—Narrower Term, RT—Related Term

Descriptions
    Catalogs
        Cultures 65

STRAINS, RICKETTSIAE

    RT Rickettsiae
    Descriptions
        Catalogs
            Cultures 66

STRESS

    NT Exercise stress
    NT Work stress
    Critical care unit person-
    nel
        Nursing practice 100

STRUCTURAL FORMULAS

    BT Formulas
    Chemicals 285
    Chemicals, European
    155
    Drugs 15, 20, 175, 285,
    371, 426, 429
    Drugs, British 55
    Drugs, new 422

STYLE MANUALS

    RT Authors' guides
    RT Copy editing
    RT Writing, medical
    Publishing, medical
        Editorial style 249
        Manuscript preparation
        249

SUBLUXATIONS

    Orthopedics
        Diagnosis 115
        Mechanism of injury 115
        Treatment 115

SUBSCRIPTION PRICES

    Journals, nursing 34

SUDDEN INFANT DEATH SYNDROME
CENTERS

    RT Death and dying
    RT Infants

Directories 203

SUICIDES

    RT Death and dying
    RT Mortality
    Medicolegal investigations
        Forensic science 292

SURGERY

    See Treatment, surgical

SURGICAL INSTRUMENTS

    See Instruments, surgical

SURGICAL INSTRUMENTS, MANU-
FACTURERS

    See Manufacturers, surgical
    instruments

SYMBOLS

    Physiology 378

SYMPTOMS

    See Signs and symptoms

SYNCOPE

    Differential diagnosis
    244

SYNDROMES

    BT Diseases
    Chromosomal anomalies
        Abstracts, literature
        69
        Atlases 69
        Etiology 69
        Natural history 69
        Signs and symptoms 69
    Diagnosis, radiologic
    368
    Differential diagnosis
    368
    Etiology 121, 217
    Inheritance 217, 368
    Metabolism 217
    Original articles
        Bibliographies 121,
        217, 368

Pathology 121, 217
Prognosis 121
Signs and symptoms 121,
  217, 368
Synonyms 121, 217
Treatment 121

SYNONYMS

  RT Dictionaries
  Chemical materials, indus-
    trial 114
  Chemicals 285, 342, 370
  Cosmetics 149
  Diseases
    Dictionaries 217
    Mendelian inheritance
      Genetics 284
  Drugs 138, 149, 285, 342
    Nursing practice 160
  Drugs, new 138, 422
  Food products 149
  Keywords 235
  Pesticides 342
  Plants, medicinal 247
  Syndromes 121, 217

SYNOVIAL JOINTS

  RT Orthopedics
  Anatomy
    Tabular data 52

SYSTEMIC DISEASES

  UF Manifestations of sys-
    temic diseases
  RT Signs and symptoms
  Cardiac manifestations
    205, 206
  Gastrointestinal manifes-
    tations 168
  Neurologic manifestations
    82
  Ocular manifestations 171
  Oral manifestations 410
    Diagnosis 399
    Epidemiology 399
    Etiology 399
    Illustrations 399
    Pathogenesis 399
    Prognosis 399
    Treatment 399
  Pulmonary manifestations
    413
  Renal manifestations 392

Skin manifestations 116

TABLES OF CONTENTS

  UF Contents, tables of
  Journals
    Clinical practice 102
    Life sciences 103

TABULAR DATA

  RT Almanacs
  RT CRC handbooks
  RT Handbooks
  RT Statistical data
  Accidents
    Signs and symptoms 286
    Treatment 286
  Algae 98
  Anatomy
    Arteries 52
    Bones 52
    Muscles 52
    Nerves 52
    Synovial joints 52
    Veins 52
  Bacteriology 98
  Barnes Hospital
    Normal laboratory values
    253
  Beverages
    Caffeine content 187
  Biochemistry
    Amino acids 94
    Buffers 94
    Carbohydrates 94
    Chromatography 94
    Ion exchange 94
    Nucleic acids 94
    Nucleotides 94
    Oligonucleotides 94
    Peptides 94
    Polypeptides 94
    Proteins 94
    Purines 94
    Pyrimidines 94
    Steroids 94
    Vitamins 94
  Biology
    Biological regulators
    48
    Biomechanics 96
    Body fluids 48
    Chemical constants 48
    Circulation 48
    Culture media 48

UF-Used For, BT-Broader Term, NT-Narrower Term, RT-Related Term

Cytology 48
Digestion 48
Electronics 96
Engineering 96
Environment, biological
  effect 48
Excretion 48
Genetics 48
Growth and development
  48
Laboratory materials 48
Mathematical constants
  48
Metabolism 48
Neurobiology 48
Nutrition 48
Parasitology 48
Physiological constants
  48
Reproduction 48
Respiration 48
Taxonomic classification
  48
Toxins, animal 48
Toxins, plant 48
Biomechanics 96
Bites and stings
  Signs and symptoms 286
  Treatment 286
Body composition 170
Body fluids 170
Body surface area
  Nomograms 418
Cancer treatment programs
  86
Chemicals 95
Chromosomal anomalies 69
Diagnostic tests
  Techniques 286
Drugs
  Pharmacology 286
Electronics 96
Elements, periodic tables
  95, 418
Engineering 96
Food composition 170
  Cholesterol content 187
  Fatty acid content 187
  Folacin content 187
  Zinc content 187
Food values
  Pediatrics 304
Fungi 98
Household equivalents 145
Infant formulas
  Content 187

Indications for use 187
Injuries
  Signs and symptoms 286
  Treatment 286
Inorganic compounds 95
Laboratory science, clini-
cal
  Bacteriology 99
  Blood banking 99
  Fungi 99
  Hematology 99
  Immunology 99
  Immunopathology 99
  Mycology 99
  Nosocomial infections
    99
  Nuclear medicine 99
  Parasitology 99
  Rickettsiology 99
  Toxicology 99
  Virology 99
Life tables 437
Mathematics 95, 170
Microbial composition
  Amino acids 98
  Carbohydrates 98
  Lipids 98
  Minerals 98
  Nucleic acids 98
  Proteins 98
Microorganisms 98
Molecular biology
  Handbooks 94
Normal laboratory values
  67, 92, 104, 105, 110,
  111, 145, 156, 172, 187,
  196, 286, 296, 351, 384,
  391, 400, 415
  Blood 77
    Nursing practice 144
  Bone marrow 77
  Nursing practice 312,
    313
  Pediatrics 192, 304
Nursing practice
Metrology 313
Posology 313
Nutrition 170
Organic compounds 95
Pediatrics
  Blood pressure 195
  Conversion formulas 195
  Growth tables 195
  Normal laboratory values
    195
  Nutrition 195

Physicians
  Licensure requirements,
    state 128
Physics 95
Poisoning
  Signs and symptoms 286
  Treatment 286
Probability 170
Protozoa 98
Radioactive isotopes 285
Recommended dietary allow-
  ances 54, 145, 400
Temperature equivalents
  145
Viruses 98
Weight, desirable 110,
  145
Weights and measures 52,
  95, 110, 145, 170, 187,
  391, 418
  Nursing practice 313

TAPES

See Audiovisual materials

TAXONOMY

RT Classification systems
  Bacteriology 39
    Microbiology 251
  Biology 48

TECHNICIANS

  Training programs
    Laboratory animal sci-
      ences 97

TECHNIQUES

See Procedures

TECHNIQUES, SURGICAL

See Treatment, surgical

TEENAGERS

See Adolescence

TELEPHONE NUMBERS

NT Tollfree telephone
    numbers
RT Addresses

RT Directories
RT Telex numbers
RT TWX numbers
Allied health sciences
  Research programs 376
Allied health sciences
  schools 261, 341
American College of Physi-
cians
  Members 45
American Medical Associa-
tion
  Committee members 14
  Officials 14
  Staff members 14
  Trustees 14
American Psychiatry Asso-
ciation
  Members 44
American Public Health
Association
  Members 46
Archives 129
Biological sciences
  schools 341
Biomedical sciences
  Research programs 376
Boards of nursing 296
Boards of pharmacy, state
  136
Burn centers 296
Buyers' guides
  Manufacturers, health
    care products, Canada
    58
Cancer protocols, experi-
mental
  Investigators 87
Cancer research institutes
  230
Cancer treatment centers
  230
Cancer treatment programs
  86
Chemical distributors 68
Congressional subcommit-
tees
  Health care 299
Consultants
  Health care 261
Dental schools 341
Dentistry
  Research programs 376
Federal information cen-
ters 129
Federal job information

centers 129
Foundations 163
Funeral service schools
  389
Governmental agencies
  151, 261, 299, 423
Hospital administrators
  123
Hospitals 58, 184, 261,
  424
  Nursing practice 317
Hospitals, United Kingdom
  268
Information centers 129
Information services 150
Information systems 150
Laboratories 424
Libraries for the blind
  129, 261
Libraries, medical 261
Libraries, research 129
Libraries, special 129
Library networks 129
Licensure
  Examination boards,
    state 424
  Licensing boards, state
    424
Manufacturers, chemicals
  68, 85
Manufacturers, drugs 136
Manufacturers, drugs, non-
  prescription 349
Manufacturers, drugs, pre-
  scription 348
Manufacturers, equipment,
  medical 263
Manufacturers, health
  care products 58
Manufacturers, laboratory
  equipment 183
Manufacturers, laboratory
  instruments 183
Manufacturers, medical de-
  vices 267
Manufacturers, medical
  products 263
Manufacturers, surgical
  instruments 387
Medical schools 1, 2,
  261, 275, 341
Medical schools, United
  Kingdom 268
Multihospital systems 184
Nursing schools 341
Organizations, dental 151

Organizations, health care
  business 184
Organizations, medical
  58, 147, 151, 261
  Publications 385
Organizations, nursing
  151
Organizations, pharmacolo-
  gy 136, 151
Organizations, scientific
  147
Patent depository librar-
  ies 129
Pediatrics
  Health care services
    297
  Mental health services
    297
  Treatment facilities
    297
Pharmacists 343
Pharmacology
  Research programs 376
Pharmacy schools 341
Physicians, United Kingdom
  268
Poison control centers 5,
  225, 246, 261, 296, 348,
  349
Public health schools 341
Publishers
  Books, in print 53, 265
  Journals 420
Research centers 375
Research institutes, for-
  eign 445
Runaway youth centers
  297
Senators and representa-
  tives 299
Specialists 126
Universities, world 445
Veterinary medicine
  Research programs 376
Veterinary medicine
  schools 341

TELEX NUMBERS

RT Telephone numbers
Cancer research institutes
  230
Cancer treatment centers
  230
Chemical distributors 68
Manufacturers, chemicals

68
Research programs   376

TEL-MED

Directories   203

TEMPERATURE EQUIVALENTS

Tabular data   145

TERATOGENIC AGENTS

RT   Adverse effects
RT   Teratology
Abstracts, literature
  Chemicals   64
  Drugs   64
  Physical factors   64
  Viruses   64
Indexes, literature
  Chemicals   64
  Drugs   64
  Physical factors   64
  Viruses   64

TERATOLOGY

RT   Birth defects
RT   Chromosomal anomalies
RT   Teratogenic agents
Genetics   270

TERMINAL CARE

See Death and dying

TERMINOLOGY

UF   Medical terminology
NT   Greek terms
NT   Latin terms
RT   Classification systems
RT   Combining forms
RT   Dictionaries
RT   Etymology
RT   Keywords
RT   Greek combining forms
RT   Greek etymology
RT   Latin combining forms
RT   Latin etymology
RT   Nomenclature
Anatomy, human   180
Health sciences   421
Medicine   421
  Abbreviations   279

Dictionaries, inverted
  235
Manuals   447

TEST REAGENTS

See Reagents

TESTING PROCEDURES

See Examinations

TESTS

NT   Assays
RT   Diagnosis, laboratory
Microbiology
  Bacteriology   251
  Formulas   35
  Fungi   251
  Procedures   35
  Rickettsiae   251
  Spirochetes   251
  Viruses   251

TEXTS

Bill of rights, dying per-
sons
  Nursing practice   438
Bill of rights, patients
6, 120
  Nursing practice   438
Bill of rights, pregnant
patients
  Nursing practice   438
Ethical codes
  Medical practice   148

THESAURI

RT   Indexes, thesauri
Allied health sciences
  262
Dentistry   262
Medicine   262
Reference books
  Indexes   162
Veterinary medicine   262

THORAX

UF   Chest
RT   Respiratory system
Diseases
  Diagnosis   173, 417

UF-Used For, BT-Broader Term, NT-Narrower Term, RT-Related Term

Pathophysiology   417
Treatment   173
Treatment, surgical   173
   Anatomy   417
   Anesthesia   417
   Postoperative care
   417
   Preoperative care   417
   Techniques   173, 417

THROAT

See Otolaryngology

THROMBOSIS

RT   Hematology
Pathology   329

TIME OF DEATH

RT   Death and dying
Medicolegal investigations
   Forensic science   292

TIMETABLES, ACADEMIC

See Academic timetables

TISSUES

See Histology

TOLLFREE TELEPHONE NUMBERS

BT   Telephone numbers
Chemical distributors   68
Manufacturers, chemicals
   68
Manufacturers, drugs   348

TOPOGRAPHY

Pathology
   Classification systems
   398

TORTS

Law
   Nursing practice   241

TOXICOLOGY

NT   Forensic toxicology
RT   Adverse effects

RT   Emergency care
RT   Poisoning
Air pollution
   Pharmacology   175
   Signs and symptoms   175
   Treatment   175
Animal toxins   48
Chemical additives
   Nutrition
      Food supply   293
Chemical materials, indus-
  trial
   Test animals
      Quantity of exposure
      114
      Route of exposure   114
Chemicals   285
   Bibliographies, annotat-
     ed   370
   Regulations   370
   Standards   370
Commercial products, chem-
  icals   85
   Emergency care   85
   First aid   85
   Signs and symptoms   85
   Treatment   85
Drugs   20, 138, 175, 285
Drugs, immunosuppressive
  73
Drugs, new   138
Drugs (treatment modality)
   Diseases
      Allergy   12
      Rheumatology   31, 414
      Veterinary medicine
      435
Heavy metals
   Chemistry   175
   Diagnosis   175
   Distribution   175
   Excretion   175
   Pharmacokinetics   175
   Sources   175
   Treatment   175
History
   Bibliographies, annotat-
     ed   264
Information sources
   Audiovisuals   225
   Data bases   225
   Graduate schools   225
   Legislation   225
   Organizations   225
   Periodical literature
   225

Reference books   225
Regulations   225
Laboratory science, clini-
cal
   Tabular data   99
Pathology
   Physiology   388
Pediatrics   439
Pesticides
   Pharmacology   175
   Signs and symptoms   175
   Treatment   175
Plants, medicinal   247
Signs and symptoms   67
Solvents
   Pharmacology   175
   Signs and symptoms   175
   Treatment   175
Treatment   67
   Drugs (treatment modali-
   ty)
      Nursing practice
         Diseases   160
Treatment, chemicals
   Cancer   79
Vitamins
   Nutrition   293

TRACHEAL INTUBATION

   Anesthesia   233

TRADE NAMES

   UF   Names, trade
   RT   Brand names
   RT   Generic names
   RT   Pharmacological names
   Chemical compounds   342
   Commercial products, chem-
   icals   85
   Drugs   15, 156, 298, 342
      Nursing practice   137,
      160
      Patient education   21
      Pediatrics   195
   Drugs, injectable   194
   Drugs, new   422
   Drugs (treatment modality)
      Oral diseases   5
   Pesticides   342

TRADEMARKS

   Chemical formulations   68
   Chemicals   285

Dentistry   216
Drugs   285

TRANSMISSION

   Communicable diseases   91,
   215, 259, 296
      Travelers   430
   Nosocomial infections   259
   Pediatrics   296
   Poisoning
      Foods   259
   Public health   259
   Sexually transmitted dis-
   eases   259
   Tropical medicine   215

TRANSPLANTATION

   RT   Treatment, surgical
   Immunology   37, 250, 360
   Liver
      Indications   132
      Techniques   132
   Organ preservation   360
   Techniques   360
   Treatment, surgical   110

TRAUMA

   See Emergency care

TRAUMA DEATHS

   RT   Death and dying
   Medicolegal investigations
      Forensic science   292

TRAVELERS

   Chemoprophylaxis   215
   Diseases
      Geographical occurrence
      430
      Modes of transmission
      430
      Warnings   430
   Health risks   430
   Malaria risks   430
   Nursing practice
      Recommendations   313
      Requirements   313
   Recommendations   354, 355
   Tropical medicine   215
   Vaccination requirements
   215, 430

TREATMENT

NT Treatment, chemicals
NT Treatment, endocrine
NT Treatment, experimental
NT Treatment, immunother-
      apy
NT Treatment, radiation
NT Treatment, surgical
 Accidents
    Pediatrics 108, 109
 Acid-base disturbances
    236
 Adverse effects
    Anesthesia, regional
      238
 Air pollution
    Toxicology 175
 Alcohol abuse
    Adolescence 109
 Birth defects 49
 Birth fractures
    Orthopedics
      Atlases 115
 Bites and stings
    Emergency care
      Nursing practice 144
    Encyclopedias 196
    Handbooks 111
    Pediatrics 109, 304
    Tabular data 286
 Burns
    Emergency care 136
    Handbooks 111
    Pediatrics 109
 Chemicals
    Poisoning 193
 Choking 105
    Emergency care 136
 Commercial products, chem-
    icals
    Poisoning 85
    Toxicology 85
 Cosmetics
    Poisoning 193, 351
 Diseases 50, 67, 73, 105,
    111, 145, 253, 286, 288,
    356
    Adolescence
      Gynecology 186
    Adrenals 57
    Aged 72
    Ambulatory medicine 358
    Animals 131
    Bile ducts 132, 133
    Blood vessels 205

Cancer 7, 61
Child psychiatry 89
Communicable diseases
  91, 223, 354, 355
    Pediatrics 224, 296,
      373
    Public health 259
    Treatment, surgical
      395
    Tropical medicine 215
Coronary artery diseases
    Nursing practice 62
Critical care
    Nursing practice 100
Dentistry, operative
    320
Dermatology 26, 116,
    256
Electrolyte disturbances
    74, 236, 372, 392
Emergency care 142,
    143, 253, 356
    Nursing practice 144,
      290
    Pediatrics 108, 192,
      252, 412
Encyclopedias 196
Encyclopedias, loose-
    leaf 81
Endocrine system 153,
    405
    Gynecology 76
Family medicine 281,
    406
Fluid disturbances 74,
    236
Gallbladder 132, 133
Gastrointestinal system
    75, 168, 169
Genetics 270, 287
Genitourinary system
    172
Genitourinary system,
    female 185
Gynecology 106, 191,
    311, 318
    Urology 185
Heart 173, 205, 206
Hematology 77, 207
Immunology 37
Kidneys 236, 372, 392
Liver 132, 133
Lungs 173
Mental illness 291
Mouth 324, 410
Nervous system 306, 408

Encyclopedias, loose-
leaf 82
Newborns 305, 382
Nosocomial infections
Public health 259
Nursing practice 242
Nutrition 293
Tropical medicine 215
Obstetrics 441
Urology 185
Ophthalmology 171, 323
Orthopedics 115,165,
254, 326, 327
Pediatrics 337
Otolaryngology 328, 411
Parasitology 168
Arthropods 83
Helminths 83
Protozoa 83
Patient care
Nursing practice 277
Patient education 21
Pediatrics 108, 109,
304, 339
Emergency care 412
Gastrointestinal sys-
tem 335
Gynecology 186
Handbooks 192
Hematology 208
Nursing practice 88
Ophthalmology 336
Orthopedics 337
Psychiatry 89, 291
Respiratory system 365,
366, 413
Rheumatology 31, 84,
414
Sexually transmitted
diseases
Public health 259
Thorax 173
Urology 57, 112
Veterinary medicine
Cats 416
Cattle 432
Dogs 416
Horses 432
Pigs 432
Sheep 432
Small animals 113
Dislocations 165
Atlases 115
Pediatrics 337
Drug abuse
Adolescence 109

Nervous system
Encyclopedias, loose-
leaf 82
Psychiatry 89
Drug interactions 135
Fracture-dislocations
Atlases 115
Fractures 165, 327
Atlases 115
Emergency care 136
Pediatrics 337
Heavy metals
Toxicology 175
Household products
Poisoning 351
Industrial hazards
Poisoning 351
Infertility
Sexual function, male
57
Injuries
Athletics 419
Genitourinary system,
female 185
Orthopedics 165
Tabular data 286
Insecticides
Poisoning 351
Malnutrition 293
Nursing care 242
Techniques
Expected outcome 294
Nursing order 294
Nutritional deficiencies
Tropical medicine 215
Oral manifestations
Systemic diseases 399
Overdose
Drugs
Nursing practice 313
Drugs, nonprescription
349
Pain
Nervous system 306
Nursing practice 63
Pesticides
Occupational diseases
319
Toxicology 175
Poisoning 351, 356
Adverse effects 105
Animals 351
Animals, marine 352
Bites and stings 193,
351
Chemicals 193

Commercial products,
  chemicals   85
Cosmetics   193, 351
Drugs   138, 193, 351
Drugs, new   138
Emergency care
  Nursing practice   144
Encyclopedias   196
Fish
  Tropical medicine   215
Food poisoning   168, 193
  Public health   259
Handbooks   111, 350
Household products   351
Industrial hazards   351
Insecticides   351
Pediatrics   108, 109,
  192, 195, 304
Plants   193, 351
  Nursing practice   144
  Tropical medicine   215
Small animals
  Veterinary medicine
  113
Snakebites
  Tropical medicine   215
Tabular data   286
Pregnancy
  Complications   266
  Nursing practice   258
Psychiatric emergencies
  89
Sexual dysfunctions
  Nursing practice   214
  Psychosomatic disorders
  89
Shock
  Emergency care 136
  Nursing practice   144
Snakebites
  Tropical medicine   215
Solvents
  Toxicology   175
Subluxations
  Atlases   115
Syndromes   121
Toxicology   67
  Air pollution   175
  Commercial products,
  chemicals   85
  Drugs (treatment modali-
  ty)
  Nursing practice
    Diseases   160
  Heavy metals   175
  Pesticides   175

    Solvents   175
  Trauma
    Emergency care   143
      Nursing practice   144

TREATMENT CENTERS

  Directories   203

TREATMENT, CHEMICALS

  BT   Treatment
  RT   Cancer protocols, ex-
         perimental
  Cancer   60, 61
    Cross resistance   79
    Dosage and administra-
      tion   79
    Investigational agents
      79
    Toxicology   79

TREATMENT, ENDOCRINE

  BT   Treatment
  Cancer   60

TREATMENT, EXPERIMENTAL

  BT   Treatment
  RT   Cancer protocols, ex-
         perimental
  RT   Cancer research insti-
         tutes
  RT   Drugs, new
  Cancer   61

TREATMENT FACILITIES

  RT   Health care services
  Directories
    Pediatrics
      Addresses   297
      Contact persons   297
      Telephone numbers
        297

TREATMENT, IMMUNOTHERAPY

  BT   Treatment
  RT   Immunology
  Cancer   60, 79
  Abdomen
    Treatment, surgical   4

TREATMENT PROGRAMS

Diseases
  Health care services
    Directories   203

TREATMENT, RADIATION

UF   Radiation therapy
BT   Treatment
  Cancer   60, 61
    Gynecology   318

TREATMENT, SURGICAL

UF   Incisions
UF   Postoperative care
UF   Preoperative care
UF   Techniques, surgical
UF   Surgery
BT   Treatment
NT   Outpatient surgery
NT   Plastic surgery
RT   Anesthesia
RT   Operating room
RT   Pathology, surgical
RT   Transplantation
  Abdomen
    Atlases
      Chemotherapy   4
      History   4
      Immunotherapy   4
      Incisions   4
      Indications   4
      Nutrition   4
      Shock   4
      Techniques   4
    Anesthesia
      Agent selection   27
      Cardiovascular system
        Diseases   417
      Equipment   27
      Patient care   27
      Pharmacology   27
      Techniques   27
      Thorax
        Diseases   417
    Atlases
      Anatomy   24
    Bibliographies
      History   42
    Diagnosis, radiologic
      Techniques   396
    Diseases
      Anesthesia   360
      Body fluids   110, 360
      Cancer   60, 61

  Cardiovascular system
    417
  Communicable diseases
    360
    Diagnosis   395
    Epidemiology   395
    Etiology   395
    Microbiology   395
    Pathogenesis   395
    Prognosis   395
    Signs and symptons
      395
    Treatment   395
    Wound infections   395
  Electrolyte disturbances
    110, 360
  Gynecology
    Complications   401
  Heart   173
  Hemostasis   360
  Indications   360
  Lungs   173
  Monitoring   360
  Nursing practice   277
  Ophthalmology   322
  Pediatrics   397
  Postoperative care   360
  Postoperative complica-
    tions   360
  Shock management   360
  Techniques   360, 415
  Thorax   173, 417
  Transfusions   360
  Face
    Anesthesia   409
    Techniques   409
  Gynecology
    Techniques   401
  Handbooks
    Anesthesia   110
    Body fluids   110
    Communicable diseases
      110
    Complications   110
    Diseases
      Complications   110
      Diagnosis   110
      Prognosis   110
      Signs and symptoms
        110
      Treatment   110
    Electrolyte disturban-
      ces   110
    Legal aspects   110
    Metabolism   110
    Nutrition   110

UF-Used For, BT-Broader Term, NT-Narrower Term, RT-Related Term

Postoperative care 110
Preoperative care 110
Shock 110
Transplantation 110
Wound healing 110
Head
  Atlases 32
Heart
  Techniques 173
History
  Bibliographies, annotat-
  ed
    Medicine 264
Hyperalimentation
  Gynecology
    Diseases 401
Indexes, literature
  History 42
Indications 322, 415
Lungs
  Techniques 173
Maxilla
  Anesthesia 409
  Techniques 409
Mouth
  Anesthesia 409
  Techniques 409
Neck
  Atlases 32
Nursing care
  Anesthesia 11
  Patient education 11
  Techniques 11
  Wound healing 11
Obstetrics
  Analgesia 321
  Anatomy 321
  Anesthesia 321
  Childbirth 321
  Postoperative care 321
  Postoperative complica-
  tions 321
  Prenatal care 321
  Preoperative care 321
  Techniques 321
Ophthalmology
  Anesthesia 322
  Diagnosis 322
  Informed consent 322
  Instrumentation 322
  Patient education 322
  Postoperative care 322
  Preoperative antibiotics
  322
  Preoperative care 322
  Preoperative cultures 322

Sutures 322
Techniques 322
Oral diseases
  Anesthesia 409
  Techniques 409
Orthopedics 56
Pediatrics
  Anesthesia 29
  Body fluid disturbances
  397
  Electrolyte disturbances
  397
  Emotional aspects 397
  History and physical ex-
  amination 397
  Infections, postopera-
  tive 397
  Parenteral nutrition
  397
  Postoperative care 397
  Preoperative care 397
  Respiratory system 397
  Techniques 397
Postoperative care 379
  Cardiovascular system
    Diseases 417
  Complications 255
  Diagnosis, radiologic
  396
  Guidelines 255
  Gynecology
    Diseases 401
  Indications 255
  Recommendations 255
  Techniques 255
  Thorax
    Diseases 417
Preoperative care 379
  Cardiovascular system
    Diseases 417
  Complications 255
  Diagnosis, radiologic
  396
  Guidelines 255
  Gynecology
    Diseases 401
  Indications 255
  Recommendations 255
  Techniques 255
  Thorax
    Diseases 417
Procedures
  Classification systems
  347
Services
  Classification systems

347
Techniques   360, 379, 415
  Alimentary tract
    Diseases   393
  Anus
    Diseases   393, 394
  Atlases   379
  Biliary ducts, extra-
    hepatic
    Diseases   393
  Cardiovascular system
    Diseases   417
  Colon
    Diseases   393, 394
  Duodenum
    Diseases   393
  Esophagus
    Diseases   393
  Eye
    Diseases   322
  Gallbladder
    Diseases   393
  Gynecology
    Diseases   401
  Liver
    Diseases   393
  Nervous system
    Diseases   306
    Trauma   306
  Orthopedics
    Amputations   56
    Arthrodesis   56
    Arthroplasty   56
    Bones   56
    Dislocations   56
    Joints   56
    Muscles   56
    Nerves   56
    Pediatrics   337
    Tendons   56
  Pancreas
    Diseases   393
  Rectum
    Diseases   393, 394
  Spleen
    Diseases   393
  Stomach
    Diseases   393
  Thorax   173
    Diseases   417
  Urology
    Diseases   57
  Thorax
    Techniques   173
  Urology
    Case studies   107

    Complications   107
    Indications   107
    Techniques   107
  Vascular diseases
    Indications   431
    Techniques   431

TRENDS

  Cancer (in U.S.)
    Statisical data   59

TRIAGE

  Emergency care
    Nursing practice   142,
    144

TROPICAL MEDICINE

  Communicable diseases
    Control   215
    Diagnosis   215
    Distribution   215
    Etiology   215
    History   215
    Pathogenesis   215
    Pathophysiology   215
    Prevention   215
    Prognosis   215
    Signs and symptoms   215
    Transmission   215
    Treatment   215
  Nutritional deficiencies
    Control   215
    Diagnosis   215
    Distribution   215
    Etiology   215
    History   215
    Pathogenesis   215
    Pathophysiology   215
    Prevention   215
    Prognosis   215
    Signs and symptoms   215
    Transmission   215
    Treatment   215
  Poisoning (of humans)
    Fish
      Diagnosis   215
      Etiology   215
      Pathophysiology   215
      Prognosis   215
      Signs and symptoms
      215
      Treatment   215
    Plants

Diagnosis 215
Etiology 215
Pathophysiology 215
Prognosis 215
Signs and symptoms
215
Treatment 215
Snakebites
Diagnosis 215
Pathogenesis 215
Pathology 215
Prevention 215
Signs and symptoms
215
Treatment 215
Travelers
Chemoprophylaxis 215
Immunizations 215

TWX NUMBERS

RT Telephone numbers
Research programs 376

ULTRASONOGRAPHY

RT Diagnosis, ultrasound
Encyclopedias, loose-leaf
81
Respiratory system 117
Techniques 404

UNDERGRADUATE SCHOOLS

RT Graduate schools
Ratings
Allied health education
schools 177
Bacteriology 177
Biochemistry 177
Biology 177
Chemistry 177
Microbiology 177
Nursing 177
Occupational therapy
177
Physical therapy 177
Premedical programs 177
Speech pathology 177

UNION LISTS

Journals 202

UNITED KINGDOM

See terms below as thesaurus
entries for detailed infor-
mation
Drugs, British 55
Drugs, European 257
Hospitals, United Kingdom
268
Journals, United Kingdom
268
Medical schools, United
Kingdom 268
Physicians, United Kingdom
268, 274

UNITS OF MEASUREMENT

See Weights and measures

UNIVERSITIES

See also Education for
listing of schools
BT Universities, world
Graduate schools
Ratings
Bacteriology 176
Biochemistry 176
Biology 176
Chemistry 176
Dental schools 176
Medical schools 176
Microbiology 176
Nursing schools 176
Pharmacy schools 176
Public health schools
176
Undergraduate programs
Ratings
Bacteriology 177
Biochemistry 177
Biology 177
Chemistry 177
Microbiology 177
Nursing 177
Occupational therapy
177
Physical therapy 177
Premedical programs
177
Speech pathology 177

UNIVERSITIES, WORLD

NT Medical schools, for-
eign
NT Universities

Directories
  Addresses 445
  Dates founded 445
  Faculty members 445
  Faculty, number of 445
  Students, number of 445
  Telephone numbers 445

UNIVERSITY PROGRAMS

NT Allied health sciences
    schools
NT Biological sciences
    schools
NT Dental schools
NT Medical schools
NT Medical schools, for-
    eign
NT Nursing schools
NT Pharmacy schools
NT Public health schools
NT Veterinary medicine
    schools
  Directories 341

URINE EXCRETION

BT Excretion
 Body fluids
  Physiology 40

UROLOGY

RT Genitourinary system
RT Genitourinary system,
    female
 Diseases
  Diagnosis 57
  Etiology 57
  Signs and symptoms 57
  Treatment 57
  Treatment, surgical
    Techniques 57
 Examination
  Instrumentation 57
  Techniques 57
 Gynecology
  Diseases
    Diagnosis 185
    Treatment 185
 Handbooks
  Diseases
    Signs and symptoms
    112
    Treatment 112
 Obstetrics

Diseases
  Diagnosis 185
  Treatment 185
 Treatment, surgical
  Case studies 107
  Complications 107
  Indications 107
  Techniques 107

U.S. COURT SYSTEM

 Law
  Nursing practice 241

U.S. GOVERNMENT AGENCIES

 See Governmental agencies

U.S. GOVERNMENT DOCUMENTS

RT Governmental agencies
 Ordering information
  Behavioral sciences 282
  Biomedicine 282
  Consumer safety 282
  Environmental health
  282
  Health sciences 282
  Hospital administration
  282
  Medicine 282
  Occupational health 282
  Patient education 282
  Vital statistics 282

U.S. GOVERNMENTAL STRUCTURE

 Law
  Nursing practice 241

U.S. JURISPRUDENCE

 Law
  Nursing practice 241

U.S. LEGISLATION

 Law
  Nursing practice 241

U.S. PHARMACOPEIAL CONVENTION

UF Pharmacopeial conven-
    tion, U.S.
 Constitution 426
 History 426

UF-Used For, BT-Broader Term, NT-Narrower Term, RT-Related Term

UTILIZATION

Health care facilities
  Statistical data   157
Health care resources
  Statistical data   204
Hospitals
  Statistical data   212

VACCINATION REQUIREMENTS

Travel   430

VACCINES

RT   Communicable diseases
  Immunizations
    Pediatrics   108

VASCULAR DISEASES

RT   Arteries
RT   Cardiovascular system
RT   Hematology
  Treatment, surgical
    Indications   431
    Techniques   431

VEINS

BT   Cardiovascular system
RT   Arteries
RT   Blood
RT   Hematology
  Anatomical tables   52,
   145, 283

VENTILATION PROCEDURES

RT   Occupational health
  Chemical materials, industrial   114

VERTIGO

Differential diagnosis
 244

VETERINARY MEDICINE

RT   Animals
RT   Veterinary medicine
      schools
  Cats
    Diseases
      Diagnosis   416

Etiology   416
Histopathology   416
Signs and symptoms
 416
Treatment   416
Physiology   416
Cattle
  Diseases
    Autopsies   432
    Control   432
    Diagnosis   432
    Etiology   432
    Pathogenesis   432
    Pathology   432
    Signs and symptoms
     432
    Treatment   432
  Diseases
    Drugs (treatment modali-
     ty)
      Contraindications   435
      Indications   435
      Physical description
       435
      Toxicology   435
      Uses   435
      Warnings   435
    Pathology   433
    Signs and symptoms   51
  Dogs
    Diseases
      Diagnosis   416
      Etiology   416
      Histopathology   416
      Signs and symptoms
       416
      Treatment   416
    Physiology   416
  Drugs
    Actions and uses   51,
     434
    Administration   434
    Adverse effects   434
    Composition   434
    Dosage and administra-
     tion   434
    Forms of distribution
     434
    Identification
      Color illustrations
       434
    Indications   434
    Manufacturers
      Addresses   434
    Warnings   434
  Encyclopedias   146

Horses
  Diseases
    Autopsies 432
    Control 432
    Diagnosis 432
    Etiology 432
    Pathogenesis 432
    Pathology 432
    Signs and symptoms
      432
    Treatment 432
Indexes, literature 218
Nomenclature
  Anatomy 309
Pigs
  Diseases
    Autopsies 432
    Control 432
    Diagnosis 432
    Etiology 432
    Pathogenesis 432
    Pathology 432
    Signs and symptoms
      432
    Treatment 432
Reference books
  Bibliographies, annotat-
    ed 201
Research programs
  Directories 376
Sheep
  Diseases
    Autopsies 432
    Control 432
    Diagnosis 432
    Etiology 432
    Pathogenesis 432
    Pathology 432
    Signs and symptoms
      432
    Treatment 432
Small animals
  Cats
    Normal laboratory val-
      ues 113
  Diseases
    Diagnosis 113
    Etiology 113
    Pathophysiology 113
    Prognosis 113
    Signs and symptoms
      113
    Treatment 113
  Dogs
    Normal laboratory val-
      ues 113

Poisoning
  Diagnosis 113
  Prognosis 113
  Signs and symptoms 113
  Treatment 113
Terminology
  Greek etymology 278
  Latin etymology 278
Thesauri 262

VETERINARY MEDICINE SCHOOLS

BT University programs
RT Veterinary medicine
  Directories
    Addresses 341
    Chairpersons 341
    Expenses 341
    Faculty, number of 341
    Programs offered 341
    Students, number of 341
    Telephone numbers 341
    University community
      341

VIDEORECORDINGS

  See Audiovisual materials

VIROLOGY

  Laboratory animal sciences
    Handbooks 97
  Laboratory science, clinical
    Tabular data
      Handbooks 99

VIRUSES

RT Communicable diseases
  Classification systems
    Animals 146
  Microbiology
    Assays 251
    Characterization 251
    Culture and isolation
      251
    Examination 251
    Identifications 251
    Interpretations 251
    Serodiagnosis 251
    Tests 251
  Nomenclature
    Animals 146
  Tabular data

UF-Used For, BT-Broader Term, NT-Narrower Term, RT-Related Term

Handbooks 98
Teratogenic agents
  Abstracts, literature
  64
  Indexes, literature 64

VISUAL SYSTEMS

  RT Ophthalmology
  Nervous system
    Encyclopedias, loose-
    leaf 82

VITAL STATISTICS, U.S.

  BT Statistical data
  BT Vital statistics, world
  NT Births, number of
  RT Death and dying
  RT Morbidity
  RT Mortality
  RT Natality
  Calculation
    Formulas 120
  Statistical data 390, 436
  U.S. government documents
    Indexes 282

VITAL STATISTICS, WORLD

  NT Vital statistics, U.S.
  Deaths
    Ages 443
    Causes of death 443
    Sexes 443
  Mortality, infant
    Causes of death 443
  Population 443

VITAMINS

  RT Foods
  RT Nutrition
  Biochemistry
    Tabular data 94
  Excretion 175
  Food sources 54, 245,
  296, 350
  History 175
  Malnutrition 293
  Nutrition
    Metabolism 293
    Requirements 293
    Toxicology 293
  Nutritional deficiencies
  293, 296, 350

Signs and symptoms 175
Pharmacokinetics 175
Physiological functions
  296
Preparations 175
Requirements 175, 296
Uses 175

VOLUNTARY HEALTH ORGANIZA-
TIONS

  BT Organizations, medical
  Addresses
    Patient education 90

WARNINGS

  UF Contraindications
  RT Adverse effects
  Diseases
    Travel 430
  Drugs
    Breast feeding 232,
    428
      Patient education 427
    Cardiovascular drugs
      Nursing practice 62
    Cross-sensitivity 428
      Patient education 427
    Drug interactions 428
      Patient education 427
    Handbooks 188
    Interferences 428
    Nursing practice 137,
    160, 312, 313
    Pediatrics
      Handbooks 195
    Pregnancy 428
      Patient education 427
    Veterinary medicine
    434, 435
  Drugs, European 257
  Drugs, new 138, 344
  Drugs, nonprescription
  190, 349
  Drugs, prescription 348
  Immunizations 253, 296,
  354
    Pediatrics 108
  Patient education
    Diseases 227
    Drugs 280

WASTE DISPOSAL

  RT Environmental health

RT   Industrial hazards
Chemical materials, industrial 114

WATER QUALITY MANAGEMENT

RT   Environmental health
Public health 259

WEIGHT, DESIRABLE

UF   Ideal weight
Handbooks 110
Tabular data 145

WEIGHTS AND MEASURES

UF   Measurement
UF   Units of measurement
NT   Atomic weights
NT   Molecular weights
RT   Height and weight
tables
RT   Mathematics
RT   Temperature equivalents
Conversion tables 95, 246
Nursing practice 313
Tabular data 52, 145,
170, 391, 418
Handbooks 110

WIFE ABUSE

See Battered women services

WITNESSES

Law
Nursing practice 241

WORK STRESS

BT   Stress
RT   Job burnout
Requirements
Nutrition 293

WORMS

See Helminths

WOUND HEALING

Treatment, surgical
Handbooks 110
Nursing care 11

WOUND INFECTIONS

Treatment, surgical 395

WOUND TREATMENT

Emergency care
Nursing practice 144

WRITERS, MEDICAL

BT   Authors
Directories 381

WRITING, MEDICAL

RT   Authors' guides
RT   Copy editing
RT   Proofreading marks
RT   Style manuals
Manuals 213
Manuscript preparation
213
Techniques 213

ZINC

Nutritional content
Foods 54, 187

About the Compilers

BARBARA SMITH SHEARER is Online Services Coordinator and Assistant Professor of Information Science at the University of South Alabama College of Medicine.

GENEVA L. BUSH is Head of the Medical Center Library and Assistant Professor of Information Science at the University of South Alabama College of Medicine.